The
American Medical Association

GUIDE TO
HEARTCARE

Revised and Updated Edition

The
American Medical Association
Home Health Library

The American Medical Association
Family Medical Guide

The American Medical Association
Handbook of First Aid and Emergency Care

The American Medical Association
Guide to BackCare—Revised and Updated Edition

The American Medical Association
Guide to HeartCare—Revised and Updated Edition

The American Medical Association
Guide to WomanCare—Revised and Updated Edition

The American Medical Association
Guide to Health and Well-Being After Fifty

The American Medical Association
Guide to Better Sleep

The
American Medical Association

GUIDE TO
HEARTCARE

Revised and Updated Edition

Developed by the
American Medical Association

MEDICAL ADVISORS

E. Grey Dimond, M.D.

Herman K. Hellerstein, M.D.

William J. Welch, M.D.

*Written by Douglas Gasner
and Elliott H. McCleary*

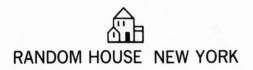

RANDOM HOUSE NEW YORK

The recommendations and information discussed in this book are appropriate in most cases. For specific information regarding your personal medical condition, the AMA suggests you see a physician. The names of organizations appearing in this book are given for informational purposes only. Their inclusion implies neither approval nor disapproval by the AMA.

Library of Congress Cataloging in Publication Data

Gasner, Douglas.
The American Medical Association
guide to heart care.
Rev. ed. of: The American Medical Association's Book
of heartcare. 1st ed. c1982.
Includes index.
1. Heart—Diseases—Prevention. I. McCleary, Elliott
Harold, 1927-   . II. Gasner, Douglas. Book of
heartcare.   III. American Medical Association. IV. Title:
V. Title: Guide to heart care.
[DNLM: 1. Cardiology—Popular works. WG 113 A5125]
RC672.G34   1984   616.1′205   83-42762
ISBN 0-394-73545-5

Manufactured in the United States of America
Second Edition
24689753

MEDICAL
ADVISORS

E. Grey Dimond, M.D., former director of the Institute of Cardiopulmonary Diseases of Scripps Clinic and Research Foundation, La Jolla, California, is Distinguished Professor of Medicine and Provost of Health Sciences at the University of Missouri in Kansas City. A graduate of the Indiana University School of Medicine (1944), he is a diplomate of the American Board of Internal Medicine and a past president of the American College of Cardiology.

A native of St. Louis, Dr. Dimond has been a Fulbright professor in the Netherlands and visiting professor at the National Heart Institute in London. He has written several books, among them *More Than Herbs and Acupuncture,* and numerous articles for professional journals. Dr. Dimond lives in Kansas City, Missouri, and Rancho Santa Fe, California.

Herman K. Hellerstein, M.D., a native of Dillonvale, Ohio, is a graduate of Case Western Reserve University School of Medicine (1941). He is currently professor of medicine at Case Western Reserve University, senior attending cardiologist at Veterans Administration Hospital in Cleveland, and a member of the medical staff of University Hospitals, also in Cleveland.

A diplomate of the American Board of Internal Medicine, Dr. Hellerstein is a former secretary of the American College of Cardiology and a former vice president of the American Heart Association. He has served as advisor to the Heart Disease Control

Program of the United States Public Health Service, as a consultant to the World Health Organization, and as a member of the Board of Directors of the Cleveland Academy of Medicine.

Dr. Hellerstein lives in Cleveland with his wife, who is a pediatrician. They have six grown children; two of their sons are medical students.

William J. Welch, M.D., is an internist with a special interest in cardiology, whose office-based practice is in New York City. A 1942 graduate of Columbia University College of Physicians and Surgeons, he is a diplomate of the American Board of Internal Medicine and a Fellow of the American College of Cardiology.

Dr. Welch is associate professor of clinical medicine at New York University Medical Center and former chief of the cardiac clinic of New York University Hospital. He is a past president of the New York [city] Heart Association, and has served as a specialist in cardiology for the New York City Health Department. He is the author of *What Happened in Between: A Doctor's Story.* Born in Eau Claire, Wisconsin, Dr. Welch lives in New York City with his wife.

American Medical Association Consumer Book Program
Thomas F. Hannon, Deputy Executive Vice President, AMA
John T. Baker, Vice President, Publishing, AMA
Charles C. Renshaw, Jr., Editorial Director, Consumer Book Program, AMA

PREFACE

Surely the most valuable asset we have, both as individuals and as a nation, is our health. Good health is the cornerstone of almost every productive human activity. And yet, all too often we squander it, either by neglecting our physical and emotional needs or by indulging in habits which are patently harmful.

In recent decades our failure to adequately maintain our health has been largely obscured by the fanfare surrounding the introduction of a host of new "wonder drugs" and an imposing array of advanced medical technology. But these innovations, despite the many benefits they have brought us, are no longer adequate, by themselves, to meet our health needs and aspirations. Something more is required; something important.

It is now clear beyond any doubt that if we wish to continue to enjoy the attributes of good health in the years ahead, the impetus will have to come from each of us, working as individuals in our own best interests. As individuals, each of us is better qualified than anyone else to act as the guardian of his or her health. By looking within ourselves and adopting prudent health habits and sensible lifestyles, we can prevent unnecessary illness, needless loss of vitality and premature old age or death.

There is, moreover, an economic urgency about all this, an urgency that affects every one of us. For a variety of reasons, medical costs have risen to unprecedented levels. Certainly one of the most effective ways the individual can help to combat this problem is to avoid what is avoidable and to help to prevent what is preventable.

These are the reasons that have motivated the American Medical Association, in collaboration with Random House, to publish this book. It is one of a series of books, to be collectively entitled the *American Medical Association Home Health Library*, which will bring you the latest, most authoritative and useful information on a wide range of health-care subjects. As doctors, we firmly believe that if you are given the facts, and the professional guidance necessary to understand and apply those facts, you will act wisely in your own behalf.

Major cardiovascular diseases are the leading cause of death in the United States, but the encouraging news is that the death rate from these diseases has declined significantly in the past thirty years. Available evidence indicates that this has been due, at least in part, to preventive care (the control of hypertension, smoking and cholesterol levels, etc.).

It is our purpose in this book to show you what researchers have found out in the area of preventive care for heart disease so that you can apply this knowledge to your own individual situation. We will also tell you about scientific advances that give new hope to people who have already suffered heart attacks, and we will show you what some of the latest medical advances in cardiovascular research portend for the future. We want you to know what your doctor and your hospital can do for you, and most important, what you can do to help yourself.

The practice of medicine is an art as well as a science, and it is thus susceptible to varying opinions regarding the exact procedures that should be followed in any individual case. Nonetheless, we are confident that the information in this book reflects the highest standards of scientific accuracy.

Let me add just one final thought: we look upon this book as an important opportunity to talk directly with you, the individual consumer of health- and medical-care services. We believe that once you are equipped with sound and balanced information, you will be able to shape a better, more fruitful life for yourself and those closest to you. That is certainly our hope.

James H. Sammons, M.D.
Executive Vice President
American Medical Association

ACKNOWLEDGMENTS

Numerous individuals have generously donated their time and expertise to the preparation of this book, and we are deeply grateful to them for their contributions. In addition to Drs. E. Grey Dimond, Herman K. Hellerstein and William J. Welch, whose guidance and counsel have been invaluable, we wish to express our thanks to the following individuals and organizations:

The American Heart Association (Dallas, Texas); Paul J. Axelrod, M.D. (Boston, Massachusetts); George Biddle (Seattle, Washington); Robert S. Bobrow, M.D. (Commack, Long Island, New York); Helen B. Brown, Ph.D. (Cleveland, Ohio); Robert B. Brown, M.D. (Seattle, Washington); Michael H. Burnham, M.D. (Los Angeles, California); William P. Castelli, M.D. (Framingham, Massachusetts); Auerlio Chaux (Los Angeles, California); Monica Chinn, R.N. (Seattle, Washington); Kim Clark, M.S.W. (Seattle, Washington); Leonard A. Cobb, M.D. (Seattle, Washington); Raye Cohen (Seattle, Washington); John J. Collins, Jr., M.D. (Boston, Massachusetts); Nelson Coon (Martha's Vineyard, Massachusetts); Kenneth M. Cooper, M.D. (Dallas, Texas); Theodore Cooper, M.D. (New York, New York); Donald W. Crawford, M.D. (Los Angeles, California); Regis DeSilva, M.D. (Boston, Massachusetts); Dolores Doehler (Des Plaines, Illinois); Claudia Dowling (New York, New York); Jane Elleson (Cleveland, Ohio); John

Farquhar, M.D. (Palo Alto, California); Marjorie and William Fix (Bellingham, Washington); Michael Foley (Seattle, Washington); Barry A. Franklin, Ph.D. (Cleveland, Ohio); Richard Frederickson (Seattle, Washington); Dan Gallion (Seattle, Washington); Walter G. Gasner, M.D. (Block Island, Rhode Island); Ray W. Gifford, Jr., M.D. (Cleveland, Ohio); Bert Green, M.D. (Seattle, Washington); Edgar Haber, M.D. (Boston, Massachusetts); Suzanne G. Haynes (Rockville, Maryland); Marie and William Hougesen (Chicago, Illinois); Howard Hunt, Ph.D. (San Diego, California); Stuart Jamieson, M.D. (Palo Alto, California); Robert Jarvik, M.D. (Salt Lake City, Utah); John Joyce (Niles, Illinois); William B. Kannel, M.D. (Framingham, Massachusetts); Ancel Keys, Ph.D. (Minneapolis, Minnesota); Duncan A. Killan, M.D. (Kansas City, Missouri); Willem J. Kolff, M.D., Ph.D. (Salt Lake City, Utah); Howard Lewis (Dallas, Texas); Bernard Lown, M.D. (Boston, Massachusetts); Shirley Mathistad (Minneapolis, Minnesota); Noel D. Nequin, M.D. (Chicago, Illinois); Barry Newcomb (Seattle, Washington); Steven Nielsen (Salt Lake City, Utah); Donald Oken, M.D. (Syracuse, New York); Donald B. Olsen, D.V.M. (Salt Lake City, Utah); Irvine H. Page, M.D. (Cleveland, Ohio); Peer Portner, Ph.D. (Oakland, California); Bruce Reitz, M.D. (Palo Alto, California); Robert L. Ringler, Ph.D. (Rockville, Maryland); Hans Selye (Montreal, Quebec, Canada); Richard B. Shekelle, Ph.D. (Chicago, Illinois); William E. Shell, M.D. (Los Angeles, California); John Simpson, M.D. (Palo Alto, California); William Snyder (Palo Alto, California); Jeremiah Stamler, M.D. (Chicago, Illinois); Frederick Stare, M.D. (Boston, Massachusetts); Kathleen B. Stitt, Ph.D. (Birmingham, Alabama); Marjorie Swain (Los Angeles, California); Charles Swencionis, Ph.D. (San Francisco, California); Edwin Traisman (Madison, Wisconsin); Gene Trobaugh, M.D. (Seattle, Washington); Robert W. Wissler, M.D. (Chicago, Illinois); Earl H. Wood, M.D., Ph.D. (Rochester, Minnesota); Peter Wood, Ph.D. (Palo Alto, California).

To C. A. Wimpfheimer and Klara Glowczewski of Random House, our sincere thanks for their knowledgeable guidance and steadfast support which were the compass points that kept our ship on course.

We also want to express our gratitude to the following members of AMA's editorial team whose creativity, skill and dedication have been so important to the quality and substance of the book: Douglas Gasner, Elliott McCleary, Jack Haesly, Leonard E. Morgan, Ralph L. Linnenburger, David LaHoda, Kathleen A. Kaye, Patricia Evilsizer of the AMA Division of Library and Archival Services, Robin Fitzpatrick, Virginia Peterson and Sophie Klim. And to Marie Moore, our deep appreciation for the meticulous care and proficiency with which she typed the manuscript.

Carole A. Fina
Managing Editor
American Medical Association
Consumer Book Program

CONTENTS

PART I

PART I

1

CAN YOU PREVENT HEART DISEASE?

"Heart disease before eighty is our own fault, not God's or Nature's will." So said the eminent cardiologist Paul Dudley White, M.D., who went on to prove that each of us holds the all important keys that can determine whether we will have heart disease or not.

Dr. White and a group of colleagues used the answers to a handful of questions about everyday living—What do you eat? Do you smoke cigarettes?—to predict with startling accuracy how many men, among a group of 490 employees of a large corporation, would develop heart disease.

In the 1930s, at the time of Dr. White's study, the art of predicting heart disease was generally frowned upon because no one knew what factors could influence the outcome. But Dr. White and his associate Menard Gertler, M.D., devised a formula for weighing the crucial elements of living that tend to bring on heart attacks. The data on smoking habits, leanness, diet and family medical history were taken into consideration. Out of the original 490 subjects, the doctors identified 32 "probables"—people whose lifestyles put them on a collision course with heart disease.

In the cold, impersonal world of medical statistics, there is a tendency to forget that human lives are at stake. But that was just the point that Dr. White was trying to make: his numbers represented living, breathing men, none of whom had any reason to suspect that a heart attack lurked in his future. In fact, at the time

Dr. White did his research, their medical records were clean—there was no indication of heart disease among any of the 490 people in the company, nor among the 32 "probables."

Yet within four years, 28 of the 32 supposedly "medically normal" men had developed heart disease. Twenty suffered heart attacks—five of them were fatal. Eight others were afflicted with angina pectoris, the painful reduction in blood supply to the heart muscle that can serve as an early warning of problems in the coronary circulation. Of the four who escaped any signs of heart disease, two were later hit by angina.

The disease that leads up to a heart attack does *not* necessarily produce any symptoms until one day when it causes angina or a full-blown attack. There is no routine test that will detect it before it does harm. Some tests on the heart can reveal dangerously constricted coronary arteries, but these are expensive, time-consuming medical procedures that are usually performed before heart surgery in instances where chest pain has become disabling and there is no other recourse.

For most people, the first sign that something is wrong within the coronary arteries is an actual heart attack. This is precisely what happened to most of the men whom Dr. White identified. They thought nothing was the matter with them. Why should they have believed otherwise? They felt fine and had no symptoms. Then, seemingly out of the blue, they suffered heart attacks. The luckier ones got some advance warning with angina or unaccustomed fatigue.

No one knows why one person will get angina and another person a heart attack. They seem to be knots on the same rope—but one of them, the actual heart attack, is further toward the end of the rope. But the average life expectancy for someone who develops angina is almost the same as that for a person who has recovered from a heart attack. In other words, no matter how heart disease first manifests itself, it should never be taken lightly.

Unlike so many other diseases that medical science has encountered, no microbes or viruses lurk behind the scenes of a heart attack. Evidence points to a slow, silent process that culminates in a shortage of blood to the heart muscle itself. It seems often to be influenced, as Dr. White found out, by the way we live—a lifestyle disease.

The increase in the number of deaths due to heart attacks corre-lates closely with the advent of labor-saving devices and the substi-tution of wheels for legs, vacuum cleaners for brooms, and fat for muscle. The mechanization of the working place, the mushroom-ing of convenience appliances in the home, and electrical refriger-ation created an environment that began to shape and intrude upon the world of flesh and blood in ways for which the human body had not been prepared.

One theory suggests that as inactivity came to be the norm and as diets became greasy and sweet, fat began adhering to the inner lining of blood-vessel walls. Slowly, over ten, twenty or thirty years, a mixture of dead and dying cells, fat and clotted blood, often followed by deposits of flinty calcium, progressively en-crusts the vascular wall, narrowing the channel and choking off the flow of blood. Such obstructions can occur anywhere in the thousands of miles of the body's arteries, impeding or shutting off some or all of the blood to the heart, the kidneys, the brain or the legs.

Leonardo da Vinci, an ardent anatomist, made reference to this arterial hardening, which he believed was related to a weakness in the arterial walls. By 1910, the year in which crystals of cholesterol were identified in the inner lining of the arteries, the disease that Da Vinci had noticed was being called arteriosclerosis, or harden-ing of the arteries. Interested researchers would—years later—detect evidence of this so-called modern disease in Egyptian mum-mies, but for the time being, in the early 1900s, it remained for some particularly astute practitioners to realize that a blockage in the coronary arteries could damage the heart.

They envisioned that a heart attack begins when a coronary artery is narrowed by abnormal deposits of fat and calcium. Then a blood clot—or thrombus, as it is called—may form on this inter-nal roughened hillock, narrowing the channel, or the damaged artery may clamp closed in a sudden spasm and shut off the flow downstream to the heart muscle. Within minutes the portion of heart muscle deprived of oxygen from its blocked artery becomes starved and its ruptured cell membranes release chemicals into the surrounding tissue. The body's distress system sends impulses to the brain, and the sensation of a heart attack—sometimes excruci-ating, sometimes not—registers its presence.

Heart attack is known by many names: *coronary thrombosis,* which suggests that the attack is caused by a clot formed in the coronary arteries; *coronary occlusion,* which suggests a blocked artery for whatever reason; or *myocardial infarction,* which is a description of the end result—the damage or death by suffocation of a portion of the heart muscle.

But by any name it is still a heart attack, and as the number of attacks rose, so did extensive heart-disease research, upon which present beliefs and recommendations are based. During the years following World War II, information on dietary and general lifestyle habits poured into research laboratories from such monumental heart-disease studies as the United States Public Health Service's project in Framingham, Massachusetts; the University of California's study of San Francisco longshoremen; the Chicago Coronary Prevention Evaluation Program; and the National Institutes of Health. Practicing physicians watched these studies with growing interest, but the data left too many unanswered questions by the early 1960s to form the basis of medical recommendations. Nevertheless, it seemed clear to many physicians that many who suffered heart attacks had certain things in common.

It was circumstantial evidence to be sure, pieced together from reports on thousands of people in the United States and around the world, but heart attacks seemed linked to high levels of cholesterol and other fats in the blood, to heredity, to high blood pressure and to cigarette smoking. Study after study confirmed the trend, and in 1964 major health organizations began recommending to the American public a diet low in calories, cholesterol and saturated fat, which, by then, many cardiologists believed would lower cholesterol and thereby reduce heart attacks, even though there was no direct proof of cause and effect.

In the same watershed year, the Surgeon General of the United States Public Health Service reported the hazards of smoking, emphasizing its contribution to lung cancer. He also confirmed that there is a significant link between smoking and heart attacks. (He reaffirmed this in his 1979 report.)

These two crucial announcements were followed by a significant drop in the rate of heart-attack deaths by the end of the 1960s. For the first time, the lifestyle that had made heart disease the number-one cause of death in the United States was changing through a combination of efforts on many fronts—in hospitals, in offices of private practitioners, and in thousands of homes across the country. The heart-attack death rate has continued to drop by 3 percent every year from 1968 through 1977, the last year for which figures have been compiled.

Commenting on this turn of events in the *New England Journal of Medicine,* Weldon J. Walker, M.D., of the Los Angeles White Memorial Medical Center, gave due credit to the improvement in coronary care, including the development of the cardiac care unit (an offshoot of the intensive care unit), new medication, and the perfection of cardiac surgery. "But," Dr. Walker wrote, "probably more important than anything doctors have done directly have been certain changes in lifestyle; do-it-yourself changes by Americans who have followed the recommendations of cardiologists, the Surgeon General, and [various health organizations]."

This was in July 1977. Experience and evidence based on more than a decade of heart-disease research convinced Dr. Walker and others like him that it is possible for many men and women to confound the odds and avoid a heart attack by adjustments—often very moderate ones—in lifestyle.

This was good news, and it began to catch on. Through the 1970s the number of adults who smoked declined, and moderation in the consumption of fats led to a decrease in the cholesterol level of the average adult in the United States. A pattern of living adopted by a continually growing number of people began making inroads into the epidemic of heart disease.

The message that a heart attack could be the final result of a lengthy disease—one that produces no symptoms until it has a virtual stranglehold on the coronary arteries—means that preventive measures should not be postponed until the first twinges of pain. Ideally, prevention should begin during childhood, when the habits that lead to health or disease are first established. A University of Iowa survey (1971–75) revealed that 5 percent of children have significantly higher than normal blood pressure for their age levels.

There is extensive and persuasive evidence that something can be done at every stage to ward off the damage that leads to heart attacks. Says one cardiologist, "I realize we still don't have all the answers regarding heart disease. But I would feel very uncomfortable about living a life that ignored all the evidence we do have. The odds would be heavily against me."

The answer to the question "Can you prevent heart disease?" may be "yes," provided that you make some (relatively painless and moderate) adjustments in your living habits and provided that the function of your cardiovascular system falls within the average range. This book will help you assess your risk of getting heart disease and it will offer you guidance on how to reduce your risk. With this information you will be able to examine your own life from the viewpoint of what is best for your heart. Even if you have neglected heart maintenance all your life, it is probably not too late now to change. Studies by the United States Public Health Service have demonstrated that middle-aged men who were heavy smokers but then gave up cigarettes cut their risk of a heart attack from three times the normal to nearly average in less than a year. A group of 635 middle-aged Swedish men with moderately high blood pressure faithfully took their prescribed medication for four years and nearly halved their heart-attack rate—to 3.6 percent, as compared to 6.9 percent for a nonmedicated control group.

If you have already had a heart attack, it might not be too late to reduce your risk of having another one. Studies seem to show that regular exercise does cut the risk of another attack.

"Seems" . . . "appears" . . . "may be" . . . By now if you are skeptical you have pounced upon the Achilles heel of the prevention question. Virtually everything you have heard about preventing heart disease, including what is written in this book, rests on circumstantial evidence. There is no irrefutable "proof" on the subject. Human beings are not identical, nor are they equally responsive to medication, advice or stress. So we cannot make hard and fast promises; we cannot give you any guarantees. It is safe to assume that even by the time you read this, some new answers—and questions—will have appeared. It is also safe to assume that if you wait until all the evidence is in, you will not benefit from what is already known.

2

HOW THE
HEART WORKS

The beat that powers a human life begins long before birth. Sixty days after conception, an intricate network of veins and arteries is visible through the transparent skin of the thimble-sized embryo. In the center of the curved inch-long form, beneath the bent-down head and folded arm buds, a throbbing streak of red marks the core of blood circulation and the central organ of the human body. Minuscule as it is, this speck of muscle is already a fully formed replica of every other human heart. For the past month, even while assuming its final form, subdividing into chambers and quintupling in size, the red cluster has been pulsing at a measured rate.

The beat of the heart arises in the myocardium itself, the specialized muscle that comprises the bulk of the organ. Unlike the muscle fibers that, for example, move limbs or cause the pupils of the eye to dilate or contract, the heart muscle is programed by its genetic code to contract and relax on its own. The prompting for the beat originates in a patch of modified muscular tissue some 25 millimeters long and 3 millimeters thick located in the upper right portion of the heart. Called the sinoatrial node, this tissue is the heart's pacemaker. It generates the electrical impulse that causes the heart muscle to contract 60 to 80 times a minute, or faster or slower depending on various conditions. The contraction of the heart depends in part on the flow of calcium into and out of each of the cells that make up the heart muscle. By regulating the flow of calcium, through the administration of specific drugs, physicians can gain control over abnormal beats and other disorders that affect the heart and its blood supply through the coronary arteries.

Within every heart-muscle cell, chemical energy from glucose, fats, and oxygen is converted into mechanical movement. Minute fibers inside the heart-muscle cells slip past one another, causing the cells' actual length to shorten. To get some idea of what is happening, hold the tips of your fingers together with your palms facing you. Now move one hand slightly upwards so just the fingertips interdigitate in checkerboard fashion. This is an approximation of the relaxed stage of the heart-muscle fibers. When energy is supplied to this system, the fibers slip farther inward past one another, just as your fingertips pass one another if you push them between your adjacent fingers.

When this muscle-fiber contraction happens in concert with millions of similar cells, it results in a heart beat. Once they have contracted, the muscle fibers return to their relaxed state, ready for another cycle. The chemical energy that supplies the driving force inside heart cells derives from the burning of a sugar called glucose in the presence of oxygen. Both these substances are carried to the heart-muscle cells by the blood. In fact, glucose and oxygen are supplied by the blood to every cell in the body to drive the internal cellular mechanisms, whether or not these mechanisms are fibers that cause contraction or something that provides the specialized function of different cells.

Before birth, the growing heart pumps an increasing volume of blood throughout the developing body. Via the umbilical cord the flow goes to and from the placenta, the "child bed" rooted in the wall of the womb. There, separated by only the thinnest of membranes, the bloodstream of mother and baby meet. The unborn baby's blood absorbs oxygen and nutrients from the mother's blood at the placenta, and in the same process discharges carbon dioxide, nitrogen and other wastes into her bloodstream for eventual removal either through the mother's kidneys or through her lungs.

At birth, with the baby's first breaths, this process ends forever and the body switches to a new system. Hormones trigger the closing of two passages which have been short-circuiting most of the blood from one side of the heart to the other, bypassing the lungs. Now and ever after, all of the heart's blood must pass through the lungs to pick up oxygen and discharge waste gases, just as food must be absorbed through the intestinal wall, and excess water drained off through the kidneys and sweat glands.

Although the shape of the human heart—more like a pear than the classical Valentine—is engineered by genetic forces, the speed at which the heart beats seems to be determined by the size of the body in general, or perhaps by the size of the heart itself. The tiny heart of a hummingbird, for example, beats 1,000 times a minute. The massive heart of an elephant lumbers at 25 beats a minute. As the weight of the average human heart increases from two thirds of an ounce in a newborn to ten and a half ounces in a 150-pound man, it enlarges to the size of an adult fist and slows at rest from 120 beats a minute to between 60 and 80. Throughout a person's adult life the weight of the heart stays about 0.44 percent of the total body weight, fluctuating by gaining or losing fatty padding as the rest of the body adds or sheds pounds.

The heart itself is suspended by ligaments in the center of the chest, between the lungs. (The beat from the powerful left chamber, called the left ventricle, reverberates most strongly on the left side of the chest, giving a person who feels his heart the impression that it is not centrally located.) Besides being guarded by the breastbone and the rib cage, the heart is contained within a tough fibrous sac known as the pericardium (*peri* = around; *cardium* = heart). Between the pericardium and the heart is a layer of lubricating fluid, which reduces the friction of the heart's beating movements within the sac. The heart muscle itself, the myocardium, is composed of millions of muscle cells woven in a thick network. This is covered on the outside with thin protective tissue known as epicardium, and on the inside, lining the hollow chambers where the blood flows, with endocardium.

The function of the heart is to propel, by means of its pumping action, enough blood at the correct pressure so that every tissue and cell in the body gets its share of this vital fluid, which carries cells, nutrients, oxygen and other substances such as hormones supplied to it by glands. Of the approximately five liters of blood in the body, 3.2 liters is plasma—a pale amber fluid which carries everything in the blood but oxygen—and 1.8 liters is cells, some 20 trillion of them, nearly all manufactured in the soft marrow in the center of bones. Some are white cells, so named to distinguish them from the oxygen-carrying red cells, although they are not really white. The white blood cells are among the body's guardians against bacterial invasion and are capable of squeezing through the walls of blood vessels to hunt down and destroy germs as well as other organisms.

The majority of blood cells are red and doughnut-shaped, and they carry oxygen to every cell in the body via the arteries. They are so small that it would take 60,000 to cover the head of a pin, and it is these cells—variously called red blood cells, corpuscles or erythrocytes (for "red cells")—that impart the characteristic red color to the blood fluid. Their return trip through the circulatory system, after giving off their oxygen in the thin-walled capillaries and taking up waste carbon dioxide, is made through the veins. The venous system carries the oxygen-depleted blood back to the heart, where it is first routed to the lungs to exchange its cargo of carbon dioxide for fresh oxygen. From the lungs the blood travels the short distance back to the heart, from which it is pumped into the arteries to complete the circulatory cycle.

The average blood cell makes a round trip through the circulatory system's arteries and veins every 60 seconds, traveling at speeds of up to 10 miles per hour when it is ejected from the heart's left ventricle into the aorta. By the end of four months it is largely worn out, its oxygen-carrying ability nearly depleted, and it begins to disintegrate. The spleen, an organ in the abdomen, filters out the spent red blood cells (it also participates in the manufacture of a variety of white blood cells called lymphocytes, which, in turn, manufacture antibodies that are capable of neutralizing bacteria and viruses and producing immunity).

The power behind the circulation of the blood comes from the pumping force of the heart. In mechanical terms, the heart actually is a double pump, two double-chambered units completely separated by an internal fibrous skeletal wall known as the septum. Each unit consists of an atrium, or collecting chamber—an entry hall—and of a ventricle, which accepts blood from the atrium and pumps it out of the heart into the arteries that carry it to the lungs and throughout the body. (See fig. #1, color insert following page 82.)

The heart and all of the 60,000 miles of blood vessels in the human body can hardly be considered separately, since they are extensions of each other, one unit—the cardiovascular (heart-vessel) system. (See fig. #2 following page 82.) Neither the healthy nor the ailing heart can be understood except in relation to the blood vessels. In fact, most heart trouble can be traced to the blood vessels, particularly the coronary arteries that nourish the heart itself. The heart is not able to absorb oxygen and nutrients from the blood that courses through its chambers. It relies for its oxygen and nourishment on the coronary arteries that branch off the aorta and penetrate the heart's muscle. Should any of the coronary arteries become blocked through disease, the blood supply to the heart will become diminished and the heart will suffer.

When Shakespeare's King Henry VI says, "My crown is in my heart, not on my head," the great bard was unerringly on the mark, both literally and figuratively. The arteries that encircle the heart bear a resemblance to a crown. Hence, in the Latin terminology of the early anatomists, they appeared to be the heart's *corona,* or crown. The name stuck, and it is within these coronary arteries—not the heart itself—that much heart disease begins.

Heart failure (a condition that results when the heart weakens and can no longer pump efficiently) results as a rule from another abnormal condition occurring in the blood vessels—hypertension, or high blood pressure. Even many electrical malfunctions of the heart, particularly the most serious rhythm disturbances, are frequently caused by impairment of arteries feeding specialized pacemaker cells in the upper part of the heart, which ordinarily coordinate the beat so that the blood flows smoothly.

With each beat the heart pumps some two and a half ounces of blood into the sweeping arch of the aorta, the main pipeline from the heart. The first branches from this vessel, near its connection to the heart, are the coronary arteries. These blood vessels carry about 5 percent of the flow—some eight ounces a minute—to feed the heart muscle with oxygen and high-energy nutrients.

It is here in these coronary arteries that the disease leading to a heart attack begins. If deposits of calcified cholesterol, known in the parlance of medical science as arteriosclerotic plaques, accumulate in these vessels, the flow of blood to the heart muscle may be reduced, sometimes to a mere trickle. Or if the coronary artery suddenly goes into spasm, with the tiny smooth muscles that ring its walls clamping down in a contraction, the blood flow also can be slowed down dangerously. If the flow stops entirely, as a consequence of arteriosclerosis or spasm alone or in combination, the heart muscle starves to death, a sequence that causes the crushing pain or discomfort of a heart attack, from which hundreds of thousands of people die every year. It is within this context that the otherwise ordinary blood vessels called coronary arteries assume such dramatic importance.

Two coronary arteries branch off the aorta as it leaves the heart. The left coronary artery runs for about an inch along the surface of the top of the heart before it divides into two branches. The other artery courses to the right and then dips to the back of the heart. These main branches, each measuring no more than five inches in length, send smaller branches into the substance of the heart muscle. Old anatomy texts compared the diameter of the main coronaries to that of a quill pen; newer descriptions compare the diameter to that of a soda straw. At any rate, the channel is about one eighth of an inch in diameter, and through it flows the blood that keeps the heart muscle alive.

Like other arteries, the walls of the coronaries consist of three layers: adventitia, media and intima. The outermost is the adventitia, a tough fibrous layer containing small nerves and a network of still smaller blood vessels (the vasa vasorum) which provides oxygen to the walls of the coronary arteries themselves.

One theory about arterial disease suggests that when deposits of cholesterol build up within arterial walls, they impede the blood vessel's own ability to nourish itself with oxygen. As a result, some of the intermediate layer of tissue (called, appropriately enough, the media) dies, adding to the obstruction in the blood vessel. In a healthy blood vessel, the media is a firm band of interwoven elastic and muscle fibers, which contribute to the rubbery feel of arteries. The elastic tissue cushions the beat of the pulse generated by the heart and permits the artery to expand and contract. The muscle fibers, in turn, contribute to the pressure within the arteries. These fibers constrict and relax on commands issued by the nervous system. Nerves carry messages in the form of electrical impulses everywhere in the body and the central nervous system, comprised of the brain and the spinal cord.

One function of the central nervous system is to maintain a

constant watch over the body's internal environment, making certain, for instance, that food gets digested properly or that the pupils of the eyes adjust to let in the right amount of light. The same is true of blood pressure. The central nervous system automatically takes care of the fine tuning by adjusting the diameter of blood vessels through the nerves that link it to the muscle fibers in the walls of the arteries. The division of the nervous system that controls such bodily functions as blood pressure without any conscious input is called the autonomic (for autonomous) nervous system, and it is divided into two parts. One turns things up, so to speak; the other settles them down. Most of the time the two divisions of the autonomic nervous system work in partnership to keep the internal environment in balance.

In helping to regulate blood pressure, for instance, signals from nerves in the autonomic nervous system adjust the muscle fibers in arteries, causing them to contract, thereby narrowing the vessels on one signal, and relax, thereby widening them on another. When an artery expands, the blood is able to move through it more easily and the pressure falls in the widened channel. Contraction has the opposite effect, narrowing the vessel and raising the pressure. This system makes adjustments in blood pressure all the time, though we are hardly aware of them. When we are nervous or when we are emotionally excited, signals from what is called the sympathetic division of the autonomic nervous system increase our blood pressure. Similarly, when we change position from lying down to standing up, the sympathetic division increases the blood pressure. When emotional excitement subsides, or when we get back into a reclining position, the parasympathetic division brings the blood pressure back down.

The innermost layer of an artery, the lining of the vessel that is in contact with the blood, is a thin sheathing of flattened cells called the intima. This lining of the coronary arteries has also been implicated in the process of arteriosclerosis. Beyond the coronary arteries, on the arch of the aorta as it sweeps upward from the heart before curving into its sharp descent through the chest and into the abdomen, are branches that carry blood outward to the arms and farther upward to the head on each side of the neck. The ascending branches are perhaps the best-known vessels in the human body after the aorta. They are the carotid arteries, which carry about 20 percent of the total circulation into the brain, and they travel side by side with the jugular veins, which drain the head of blood.

If the carotids or any of their branches become clogged with arteriosclerotic plaques, the blood flow to the brain decreases, and in some instances where the blockage is severe enough, brain cells succumb to the shortage of oxygen. The first signs that the brain is affected by the same process that can choke off a coronary artery are various muscular weaknesses confined to one side of the body, a tendency to become forgetful or confused and even a brief period of blindness. In the heart, this sort of oxygen depletion can set off a heart attack; when it happens in the brain, it is known as a stroke. Strokes can sometimes be prevented by surgery that cleans out the obstructed portion of a carotid artery in the neck. The first such carotid endarterectomy was performed successfully in 1953 by Michael DeBakey, M.D., and is now standard procedure in many hospitals around the world. More recently, obstructions of important arteries within the head have been bypassed to prevent stroke, and a similar operation has been devised to bypass obstructions within coronary arteries.

About an inch or so beneath the ear, on either side of the head, there is a slight but remarkable bulge in the carotids, an enlargement that baffled anatomists for centuries because the bulge contains tissue that does not seem to belong inside a blood vessel. It was not until the twentieth century that the details of this curious carotid tissue were worked out, and the finished puzzle proved very revealing. The bulges—or sinuses, as they are now called—contain specialized chemical and pressure receptors. These receptors continually monitor the oxygen content of the blood and the pressure at which it is pumped.

The aorta, in its descent through the abdomen, sends branches to the stomach, liver, spleen, kidneys and intestines before splitting into two smaller, equal channels. These are the right and left iliac arteries, one for each leg. If we follow the flow of blood through any artery, either the branches that supply major organs with oxygen or those that supply the limbs, the same pattern repeats itself: the artery branches into many smaller vessels, which in turn split into smaller and smaller conduits. The narrowest of these are capillaries. They are so fine that red blood cells must proceed single file and even bend on themselves to pass through. It is within the capillaries that the exchanges between blood and cells take place. Oxygen molecules diffuse through the gossamer-like capillary walls into the cells everywhere in the body. At the same time, molecules of carbon dioxide, released by the cells, diffuse into the plasma and attach themselves to the iron-and-protein hemoglobin molecules that make up red blood cells. Other wastes from the cells also diffuse into the bloodstream, while various nutrients are transmitted from the blood to the cells for fuel.

As the red blood cells exchange oxygen for carbon dioxide, they gradually turn color, imparting a bluish tint to the bloodstream for its return trip to the heart through the veins. Capillaries, in effect, connect small arteries to small veins. Small veins connect with larger and larger ones, finally merging into the inferior (or lower) vena cava, which brings blood from the lower parts of the body back to the heart, and the superior vena cava, which brings blood from the head, arms and chest back to the heart.

The oxygen-depleted bluish blood from these veins flows into the right atrium of the heart. As the right atrium fills, the sinoatrial node or pacemaker in the upper-portion of this chamber fires an electrical impulse that is conducted by the adjacent heart-muscle cells down and across the top of the heart to initiate the wavelike contraction, or beat, of the upper two chambers. For the heart to beat properly, it cannot all beat at once, for it has to route the blood through the four chambers in a correct sequence. To accomplish this, the upper chambers beat a fraction of a second before the bottom chambers.

This top-chamber contraction propels blood from the right atrium through the three triangular leaves of the tricuspid valve, which gape as blood rushes down into the right ventricle. The heart has two valves that separate the atria and the ventricles. The tricuspid valve, just mentioned, separates the right atrium from the right ventricle. The mitral valve separates the left atrium from the left ventricle. Additionally, there are two other valves—the aortic and pulmonary valves—located at the exits of the left and right ventricles. The reason for all of them is to keep the blood flowing in the correct direction through the heart.

While the tricuspid and mitral valves permit free flow of the blood from the atria to the ventricles, they snap shut to prevent the blood from flowing back into the atria when the ventricles contract. Similarly, the aortic and the pulmonary valves allow the blood to flow into the aorta and the pulmonary artery, respectively, but they too shut to prevent any backflow when the ventricles relax. This one-way system of valves is crucial for good circulation.

A fraction of a second after the pacemaker fires, the wave of natural electricity reaches the atrioventricular node (a nerve-muscle bundle similar to the first pacemaker but located in the wall between the two ventricles), and it sparks an undulating contraction in the tapering, thickly muscular chambers of the lower heart. The contraction of the right ventricle propels the still bluish, oxygen-depleted blood through the only path open to it, the crescent-shaped pulmonary valve, which leads out of the heart into an artery that branches into the lungs.

The blood, however, does not flow into the lungs like air into a balloon. Instead it remains in the blood vessels that branch inside the lungs into a vastly intricate web of capillaries. If opened up and spread apart, this capillary network in the lungs would cover an incredible 16 acres of surface space. These capillaries weave and bend through 700 million air sacs, which are the essence of the lungs. It is within the air sacs that the capillaries exchange waste carbon dioxide for fresh oxygen. When oxygen is captured by the red blood cells within the capillaries of the lungs, the color of the blood is transformed into a flaming crimson.

The blood reoxygenated in the lungs flows quickly back to the heart, entering through the left atrium. Now, on the final leg of its cyclical journey, the blood rushes through the two-leafed mitral valve, separating the left two chambers, and plunges into the left ventricle, which pumps it out into the great arch of the aorta for distribution to all parts of the body.

It is a majestic swooshing, swirling tumult, a miniature Grand Canyon cascade that in the actual choreography of the heart takes place in the tick of a clock, with the left and right sides of the heart synchronizing in perfect harmony, both atria filling simultaneously and both ventricles pumping a mere flicker later.

The sound of the pumping heart, muffled by muscle, glistening membranes (that encase and suspend the heart in the center of the chest), and bone and skin, is the repetitive tympanic *"lub-dub"* that reverberates from the closing of the valves: *"lub"* as the tricuspid and mitral valves snap shut in the contraction (or systole) phase, *"dub"* as valves leading to the pulmonary artery and to the aorta close at the beginning of the filling (or diastole) phase.

In essence, then, the task of the right side of the heart is to accept bluish, carbon-dioxide-laden blood returning from its circuit through the body and push it into the lungs, while the job of the left side of the heart is to accept the refreshed blood from the lungs and pump it to the rest of the body. Because of this larger task, the left ventricle has three times as much muscle as the right; it is the "heart of the heart."

The rhythm of the heart's contractions, the pace and power of its beat, are influenced by impulses that travel along nerves from the brain and the spinal cord to the heart. In ancient times it was widely believed that the fourth finger of the left hand acted as a conduit to carry factors from the outside world to influence the heart. Spirits supposedly could shuttle along this route to convey messages to the heart, and in the other direction, from the heart through the finger to the outside world. It was a convenient path, to say the least, and it was put to use in numerous rituals.

Priests discovered that a gold band placed around the path could bind two hearts, and so the fourth finger of the left hand was consecrated to carry the wedding ring. Not to be outdone, Greek physicians carried the ritual a step further and adapted the pathway for their own purposes. They would plunge the hallowed finger into their nostrums, using it to stir their medicinal mixtures in the misguided belief that anything noxious in the concoction would communicate its presence by causing a palpitation of the heart. They were slightly off track, off course, but that did not stop a host of superstitions from taking root in the fertile imagery that surrounded the "healing finger," as it came to be known. Medieval folklorists claimed its touch could cure warts or heal wounds. It could also impart its salutary powers to the wedding ring, which then could be rubbed over the body, it was claimed, to alleviate any manner of ailment.

As could be expected, early anatomists sought long and hard for the elusive, magical conduit to the heart in hopes of extricating its powers for their own designs, but alas, it eluded their grasp. To be sure, they encountered nerves and arteries, but no direct channel to the mighty organ itself. Along the way, though, they solved some intriguing mysteries about the heart and straightened out a few legendary misconceptions. It turns out that the original advocates of the "fourth-finger theory" had the right idea; they were off target only by a yard or so.

The conduit to the heart is not in the fourth finger, but in the brain in a region known as the hypothalamus. Through a series of interconnections with glands elsewhere in the body, the hypothalamus coordinates a chain of hormonal messages that allows the heart to respond almost instantaneously to external events and internal emotions. From messages fed to it by the bloodstream and nervous system, the heart is kept in constant contact with the rest of the body, and from information gathered by the five senses, it is kept abreast of the outside world.

A change in the body's temperature, for instance, produces a concomitant change in the heart rate, as does a change in muscular activity, or an emotional stress or an improperly functioning thyroid gland. External stimulants, such as the caffeine in coffee, tea, chocolate and colas, can similarly spur the heart to beat faster. In fact, stimulants or fatigue, emotional stress, fever and various chemical disturbances within the body can also produce irregularities of the heartbeat, usually as one or more premature beats, a second beat piled atop the previous beat so they are sensed as one. It is experienced as a "skipped beat" and it momentarily throws the heart's rhythm out of sync, impairing the smooth flow of blood through the organ's four chambers. The heart ordinarily adjusts, getting back in step, so to speak, during the next few beats, but if the problem constantly recurs, rest or withdrawal of the offending stimulant may be necessary to correct the rhythm problem.

The cardiac regulatory center in the brain achieves its many-tentacled and delicate control of the heart and blood pressure through a combination of nerve impulses and hormonal messages that can reach far into the heart itself to override the automatic pacemaker and reset the rhythm and force of the beat. The main control circuitry between the brain and the heart consists of the two nerve pathways of the autonomic nervous system (mentioned earlier in this chapter in the context of controlling the blood pressure). The sympathetic nervous system stimulates the heart to beat faster; the parasympathetic system slows it down. If the connections are severed, in the case of heart surgery or in the dramatic case of heart transplantation, the heart will be unable to respond to directions from higher nerve centers, but it will continue to beat rhythmically to the sound, in effect, of its own drummer, the sinoatrial node, that remarkable source of the heart's pace.

Around the mid-1850s, some thirty years after a French physician named René Théophile Hyacinthe Laennec invented the stethoscope to listen to heart and chest sounds, a pair of German researchers made the startling discovery that sound was not the only thing emanating from the heart. Along with each *lub-dub*, they found, the heart releases a jolt of electricity. What they detected is, in fact, the impulse from the sinoatrial node as it is being conducted through the heart to stimulate the muscular contraction. Within another thirty years, the electrocardiogram (ECG) was born. This device simply captures the heart's electrical impulse as it is discharged and records it on a piece of paper or on a fluorescent screen. This impulse is not interrupted during an ECG recording, so the device is perfectly harmless. In fact, the machine does not interfere with any of the body's functions; it simply records the electrical echo of the beat as it is transmitted upward through the skin. But from the sharp, needlelike peaks and precipitous valleys and undulations of an ECG tracing, physicians can detect heart trouble ranging from rhythm disturbances to heart attack. If there is nothing wrong with the heart, the ECG record shows that also.

The standard ECG strip that a cardiologist runs off on his office machine during a medical checkup contains valuable information about the heart: how it is performing, or at least how it was performing at the time of the test. Sometimes the ECG strip shows minor irregularities that reflect individual variations in heart rhythm and rate. This strip will form part of the patient's medical record, and the cardiologist will be able to compare it with future ECG recordings to determine if there have been any changes.

The ECG strip alone, though, is not a crystal ball and it cannot be used, by itself, to predict the heart's future. Nor, on the other hand, is it as mysterious as it looks at first glance, with its spikes and curves. Each set of waves represents a complete heartbeat cycle. The first blip is the sinoatrial node firing. The next large peak is the impulse coursing through the left and right ventricles, which corresponds with ventricular contraction (systole). Then comes the recovery period for recharging the system when the heart's atria refill (diastole), and the beat repeats itself with a similar electrical display.

Any irregularities or abnormalities in the way the electrical impulses are conducted through the heart to synchronize the normal rhythm are known as arrhythmias, and they are reflected on the ECG record. By looking at an ECG strip, a physician can tell if the heart is beating too slowly or too quickly, or whether it is skipping beats or bunching them together or not beating effectively at all. Sometimes a spot or focus of irritated heart muscle— from a heart attack or infection of the heart muscle itself—will set off an electrical discharge outside the normal conduction pathway, but still inside the heart muscle, and an out-of-sequence beat will be triggered. If such abnormal discharges occur during an ECG test, they will appear on the record, and the physician will be alerted to the problem.

Depending on where in the cycle this abnormal discharge occurs, the physician can determine which of the heart's chambers is probably affected. The atria may beat too quickly or too slowly, and so may the ventricles; perhaps some beats will not get through to the ventricles each time. The ECG will detect all of these problems. The variety and pattern of cardiac arrhythmias are almost a medical subspecialty in itself, and reading the ECG strip and determining what is wrong from it takes practice and skill. Many of the arrhythmias that are detected by an ECG can be treated with drugs or electrical countershock (delivered through an instrument called a defibrillator, which is essentially a set of metallic paddles connected to an electrical source; the paddles feed a jolt of electricity into the heart, breaking up the abnormal electrical discharge and allowing the heart's own natural pathway to restore the smooth flow of current through the chambers), and sometimes by the insertion of an artificial pacemaker, which takes over the duties of the internal pacemaker.

The most dangerous arrhythmias affect the lower chambers of the heart, the ventricles. One such arrhythmia is called ventricular fibrillation, and it is a true medical emergency that can quickly progress to a condition that is known all too ominously as cardiac arrest. In ventricular fibrillation, the ventricles twitch helplessly in a rapid, uncoordinated beat that some surgeons say has the feel of a bag of worms. As disagreeable as this description sounds, it does justice to the catastrophic predicament that the heart is in when it is undergoing ventricular fibrillation. Within seconds after this arrhythmia has begun, the effects of no blood being pumped from the heart—for that is what happens—take their toll on the rest of the body. The pulse disappears, the blood pressure drops to an undetectable level, breathing stops, and consciousness flutters away into shadows and darkness. The brain can survive only three to six minutes without fresh oxygen before its cells suffer irreversible damage. Without immediate resuscitation in the hospital or, if the attack takes place outside the hospital, cardiopulmonary resuscitation by a person trained in mouth-to-mouth breathing and external cardiac massage, the victim can become another statistic in the mounting toll of sudden-death cardiac arrest. Of the 650,000 lives claimed by heart attacks in 1980, 400,000 of those people never made it to the hospital because they failed to recognize the symptoms in time and call for help.

Nearly all of the pieces and parts that keep the heart functioning smoothly and effectively are vulnerable to disease, either directly or indirectly. One or another of the coronary arteries can be plugged by cholesterol-laden clogs. This can starve a section of heart muscle of its blood supply, and a heart attack may ensue. Bacteria or even normal wear and tear can damage the electrical conduction system in the heart, throwing off the rhythm and causing dizziness or fatigue associated with poor circulation through the heart. The valves themselves and the special muscles that hold them in place can be damaged in a heart attack or by infection, and the valves can leak, causing the heart to work harder and harder to pump blood, and eventually wearing down even the strong muscle of the left ventricle until it is so weakened that it can no longer pump effectively.

As parts of the heart that nature designed to keep the organ working well fall victim to disease and discord, the whole heart and often most of the rest of the body suffer. The trick is to keep the components of the heart in good shape. For most of us, this means keeping the coronary arteries free of disease. But what causes them to clog up? How can it be prevented? How is it recognized when it happens? What are the symptoms? The answers to these questions, which begin with the next chapter, can mean the difference between life and death, for heart disease is the world's leading killer, and you owe it to yourself to learn what you can do about it and to take certain precautions which are clearly explained in succeeding chapters. It is the most up-to-date information from the most authoritative sources.

3

WILL YOU HAVE A HEART ATTACK?

On January 24, 1975, at a meeting of heart specialists from medical centers around the country, statistical evidence was presented which showed that the destiny of the human heart could be changed.

On that day, after a decade of mounting circumstantial evidence on the benefits of a heart-saving lifestyle, the death rate from heart attacks was announced to be on a downslide for the first time in this century. If it was a historic occasion, on the level of the discovery of antibiotics or a prevention for polio, it went largely unnoticed. Statistics, after all, are not nearly as palpable as a hypodermic needle.

No one knows exactly when the condition that we now call heart attack began claiming its toll of human lives, but it was not diagnosed with certainty until 1912, when James B. Herrick, M.D., a Chicago physician, published his account of sudden coronary artery obstruction in the *Journal of the American Medical Association*. Word of the condition and the process by which arteries of the heart can become clogged to cause the attack spread throughout the medical community. Within three decades after Herrick's article, heart attack had established its infamous reputation.

More than a million Americans will suffer heart attacks or develop angina for the first time this year. At this moment, most of them do not know that they are headed for trouble—or worse. You or somebody you know may be one of them. In fact, there

Leading causes of death

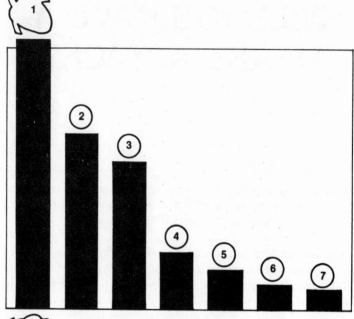

 1   Major Cardiovascular diseases

(2)   Cancer

(3)   Cerebrovascular diseases

(4)   Accidents

(5)   Influenza and pneumonia

(6)   Diabetes Mellitus

(7)   Cirrhosis of the liver

Source: National Center for Health Statistics, U.S. Department of Health, Education, and Welfare.

is a very high probability that this is so—if not this year, then the next, or the year after. Heart disease will continue progressing, and heart attacks will continue happening "out of the blue" unless you do something to change your own situation—your own risk —and if possible, the risk of those closest to you. This applies to everybody, not just middle-aged men, who have been the traditional target of heart attacks.

In the past, women have seemed less susceptible than men to such problems. Female hormones, it was felt, protected them against arteriosclerosis and heart attack, at least until menopause. But that view is changing on the basis of newer evidence. And the favorable odds—odds that made it five times less likely for women between ages thirty-five and fifty-five to die of a heart attack, compared to men—are shrinking.

The change has come about because increasing numbers of women are smoking, and smoking cigarettes is a leading cause of heart disease. The warning on the side panel of cigarette packages is almost universally taken to mean cancer, to which cigarettes are strongly linked. But that is not the whole story. The nicotine in smoke makes the heart beat faster and more strongly, while the gases in that same inhaled smoke deprive the heart of oxygen. At the same time, blood vessels throughout the body constrict, and blood pressure rises—all from a few puffs on a cigarette. Simply put, there is no doubt that smoking intensifies coronary-artery disease in both sexes.

Smoking, though, is not the only reason why women are becoming more susceptible to heart disease. Oral contraceptives, particularly if they are used by women over forty, increase the risk. Women who take the pill *and* smoke are eight times as vulnerable to heart attack as women who do neither. The mechanism by which the pill increases the risk of heart attack when it is combined with cigarette smoking may have something to do with the way the blood clots. A blood clot in a coronary artery can trigger a heart attack. If both smoking and birth-control pills affect the cardiovascular system, as they are known to do, it is conceivable that in combination their effects would be enhanced to the detriment of the heart. That, in any case, is what statistics have shown.

As Dr. White found out, the risk of your getting heart disease goes hand in hand with certain things you do, with certain habits you may take for granted. The list of risk factors is not endless. No one is asking you to give up everything you enjoy or to change your entire way of life. There are only a few risk factors about which you need to know. They are: your age, heredity, weight, the cholesterol in your blood, your blood pressure, your sex, and your smoking and exercise habits.

The roots of the risk concept can be traced back to 1947, when the United States Public Health Service, alarmed by the sheer number of heart attacks occurring in the country, undertook to determine the factors influencing the development of heart disease. At that time, knowledge about heart disease was based principally on studies of people who were already suffering from chest pain or recovering from heart attacks. It was known that certain things in their backgrounds were similar, but this was not sufficient proof. The only way to get the necessary evidence would be to devise a plan to study a typical sample of the United States population over a generation, to analyze each participant's heredity, characteristics and living habits, and thereby discover why some people get heart disease and others do not.

It was an awesome task, but the directors of the Public Health Service decided that they had no choice if they were to find out what was behind the epidemic of heart disease. After months of preliminary work, the investigators charged with the task of finding a cross section of the United States population chose Framingham, Massachusetts, a peaceful, pleasant industrial center twenty-one miles west of Boston, as their typical American town.

The Framingham Study, as it came to be known, would involve the National Heart Institute, Harvard Medical School and the Boston University Medical Center. It became the largest, best documented and most talked about single study of heart disease in the world. But at its inception no one knew that, least of all the approximately 5,000 men and women, none younger than thirty or older than sixty-two, who were enlisted out of Framingham's 28,000 residents as the study subjects.

"Study subjects." It is a term that removes the personal framework, much as statistics and risk factors do, and allows researchers to be objective. Yet these are real people, men and women who agreed to submit to interviews and medical examinations for as long as the study lasted, and we owe them a great debt because the major risk factors for heart disease were worked out on the basis of evidence gathered from their lives—evidence that is still being gathered today, for the Framingham Study continues.

As the data from the first two decades of physical examinations were compiled, computers joined the task of analyzing and comparing the medical and lifestyle histories of the study subjects. Some surprising trends started to emerge:

- A man whose blood pressure during the contraction, or systolic, phase of his heartbeat is above 150 faces more than twice the risk of heart attack as a man whose blood pressure is under 120.
- A man who smokes more than a pack of cigarettes a day has nearly twice the risk of heart attack as a man who does not smoke.
- A man with a serum (blood) cholesterol measurement of 250 or above has three times the risk of heart attack as a man with a cholesterol level below 194.

If a combination of the three factors—smoking, high blood pressure and elevated cholesterol—is present in the same person, the risk of heart attack is greater than the sum of the individual risks. Thus, a man who has elevated cholesterol and high blood pressure will have much more than five times the risk of heart attack as a man who has neither.

On the weight of these findings, Thomas R. Dawber, M.D., the principal architect of the Framingham Study, announced that high blood pressure, elevated cholesterol and cigarette smoking—the "big three"—stand out as the most important factors in the development of coronary heart disease. "All these," he noted, "are subject to change in a favorable direction by diet, drugs, and the willingness of the individual to stop smoking."

It was compelling evidence, but it did not stop there. The Framingham Study, and others similar to it in Evans County, Georgia; Albany, New York; Los Angeles, California; and Tecumseh, Michigan, identified other culprits lurking in the shadows of heart disease. While the "big three" remain predominant, such factors as your sex, obesity, a family history of heart disease, a sedentary lifestyle and stress all appear to play a role in the development of heart disease. Although you cannot, obviously, change your heredity or your sex, these factors should be heeded because they may increase your vulnerability to heart disease, especially if you have one or more of the "big three" risk factors.

One of the first things researchers who studied heart disease noted was, naturally, the most obvious fact—namely, that deaths from heart attacks increase with age. But just as obviously, there were exceptions. Some people live to be a hundred without a sign of heart trouble. Thus, scientists came to the conclusion that heart disease is not an inevitable result of aging. Hereditary factors may indeed play a part in protecting you from heart disease or increasing your susceptibility to it, but they do not entirely preordain your fate.

If your father or mother died of a heart attack at age fifty, you need not resign yourself to a similar end. Nevertheless, a tendency does exist for heart disease to run in families. If, for example, you are a man under age fifty-five and your father, brother or grandfather suffered a heart attack before reaching age sixty-five, you have five times the normal risk of repeating your relative's experience. If your sister, mother or grandmother suffered a heart attack before reaching age sixty-five, you—and this time "you" can be a man or a woman—have seven times the normal risk for your sex. The reason for this increased risk has to do with incompletely understood genetic factors and their interplay with environmental factors.

Fortunately, these odds can be altered, for they are only partially due to heredity. Researchers who patiently analyzed the statistics on families found that genes were not the only things passed from parents to children. Habits of diet, exercise and coping with the stress of life also run in families. And it is these habits which can be changed to alter the odds.

Mild obesity, although not as dangerous as was once thought, tends to run in families and contributes to high blood pressure, which, in turn, contributes to heart disease. It is, admittedly, a complicated trail of associations, but it is this type of medical sleuthing that produced success in the battle to stem the tide of heart disease. After the Framingham investigators had uncovered the fact that a 10 percent increase in weight is accompanied by an increase of 6.5 points in blood pressure and 12.5 points in cholesterol, the study's director computed that "if everyone in Framingham had maintained his or her ideal weight, there would have been 25 percent fewer heart attacks at any age and in either sex."

The Framingham evidence on exercise is not as conclusive, but it shed light on a previously little-known relationship between physical activity and cholesterol. It had been well established that reasonable exercise improves the efficiency of the human heart, benefits circulation and increases one's ability to perform physical effort and take part in recreation without strain. Our bodies tell us that exercise is good—we feel better both mentally and physically after exercising. But does it actually reduce our chances of contracting heart disease?

On the surface, it seemed likely that exercise could help, but the evidence to prove the point was scanty. There were simply too many other factors involved in heart disease, and exercise did not seem to swing the balance. Then came an unexpected break. A natural substance found in the blood appeared to be capable of protecting the body against arteriosclerosis, and this substance could be increased by exercise.

The pieces of the puzzle began falling together after two normal substances had been discovered in the blood. Both of them were found to be involved in carrying cholesterol throughout the body. One, a low-density lipoprotein (LDL), deposits cholesterol in blood vessels where it can eventually build up to clog the artery with arteriosclerotic debris. The other is a high-density lipoprotein (HDL); it acts to speed the removal of cholesterol from the walls of arteries and carry it to the liver, where it is harmlessly metabolized.

More than a decade of testing for HDL in the blood of the study subjects led Framingham investigators to the irresistible conclusion that high HDL levels are accompanied by improved resistance to heart attack. And subsequent studies elsewhere showed that the HDL levels could be raised by physical activity.

It was a roundabout discovery, typical of the difficulty in extracting information on the cause and prevention of heart disease, but the role of exercise in preventing heart disease was finally on sound, scientific ground.

Regular exercise, apparently, leads to other benefits as well, and one of the more popularized of these is the release of stress. Studies at the University of Wisconsin, the University of Virginia and Case Western Reserve University, and from Fred Heinzelmann, Department of Justice, Washington, D.C., all showed that regular exercise, such as jogging, alleviates feelings of worthlessness, improves self-image and instills a feeling of achievement.

John H. Greist, M.D., a psychiatrist who conducted the Wisconsin study, concluded that jogging worked as well as or better than psychotherapy in relieving depression, and Fred Heinzelmann reported that the formerly sedentary men in his exercise program were more energetic, felt better, needed less sleep and were more productive at work than they had been prior to the program.

The stress of ordinary everyday living has been implicated in many of the psychological conditions that exercise helps to alleviate. Indeed, the way we cope with stress may make a difference in our susceptibility to a variety of physical disorders, including heart disease.

Some evidence suggests that aggressive, hard-driving people are more prone to heart disease than easygoing types who do not react as dramatically to stress. There is also ample laboratory documentation, summarized by James C. Buell, M.D., and Robert S. Eliot, M.D., in the *Journal of the American Medical Association* in 1979, that indisputably—to use their word—links stress to accelerated arteriosclerosis and heart attack. If some physicians are still waiting for an adequate method to measure subjective feeling about stress, others are convinced from their own observations that the direction is clear, and that stress plays a role in heart disease.

According to the psychologist James J. Lynch, Ph.D., a specialist in psychosomatic disease at the University of Maryland School of Medicine, loneliness is also a factor. Individuals who live alone, says Lynch in his book, *The Broken Heart,* may be especially vulnerable to stress and anxiety because they "lack the comfort of another human being." And life-insurance-company statistics show that single, widowed, divorced or separated men and women are twice as likely to die from coronary disease as their married counterparts.

Whether loneliness affected some women in the Framingham Study is difficult to know, since it was not one of the risk factors that was assessed. In all likelihood it had some bearing on the fact that women who were married to heart-attack victims had double the heart-attack rate of women married to men who were not afflicted. It is also possible, the investigators speculated, that like tends to marry like. But some of the blame has to be placed on shared eating and living habits that contribute to, or protect against, heart disease.

It is a myth that women do not have heart attacks. They do— but their attacks occur later in life. Women tend to be resistant to heart disease, apparently from the protective influence of the female hormone estrogen, although such a conclusion is being challenged. Several years ago a large number of Chicago men who had suffered heart attacks were given regular doses of estrogen in an effort to find out if it could protect them from further heart disease. Besides distressing side effects—including loss of libido and swollen, tender breasts—the treatment backfired and the experiment was aborted when the rate of recurrent heart attacks actually increased.

A woman's risk of heart attack gradually increases with the decline of female hormones during and after menopause. But other factors can accelerate her vulnerability. When a woman over age forty smokes *and* takes oral contraceptives, she increases the risk of heart attack manifold, as mentioned earlier. Yet the facts and figures regarding the pill keep changing. Most oral contraceptives, for example, now have less estrogen than those used in the older studies that implicated them as a health threat (and some of the progestin "mini-pills" have no estrogen). And what's more, most of the warnings about the pill relate to blood clots and strokes, not heart attacks. So there is reason for confusion on this issue.

In an attempt to clarify the situation, an editorial in the *Journal of the American Medical Association* summarized the research data and advised that any woman taking the pill should be examined periodically for an increase in cholesterol, blood pressure and blood sugar, any of which can be elevated during oral-contraceptive use. If a significant increase occurs, it is time to consider another method of birth control—the levels will ordinarily fall back to normal when oral-contraceptive use is discontinued.

Converging evidence from all the studies supported one basic fact: people could alter their own chances of developing heart disease by changing certain habits or risk factors.

To test the core of this hypothesis, the National Institutes of Health began, in 1972, a massive experiment to ascertain what would happen if a large group of people modified their serum-cholesterol and blood-pressure levels and their cigarette smoking habits. Would the results be a reduction in the coronary death rate over a number of years?

The experiment, sponsored by the National Heart, Lung and Blood Institute, was designed to answer the nagging question about cause and effect.

Groundwork began with the selection of 12,866 men between the ages of thirty-five and fifty-seven who, because of smoking habits and high serum-cholesterol and blood-pressure levels, had an increased risk of developing coronary heart disease, even though they had no clinical evidence of the disease.

The study, known as MRFIT—for Multiple Risk Factor Intervention Trial—was restricted to men because they have a much higher risk of heart attack at an early age than women.

Half of the men were assigned to a special group that would receive frequent individual attention by a MRFIT intervention team. Depending on their particular combination of risk factors, the men in this group were counseled to quit smoking; they were encouraged to lower their serum cholesterol level through recommended changes in their eating patterns; and they received drugs to help reduce their blood pressure if weight reduction plans failed.

All the other men in the study were assigned to a "usual-care" group and were referred to their personal physicians or other community medical facilities for individual treatment of their risk factors.

It was anticipated from the beginning that the men in the usual-care group would serve as controls against which to measure the results from the special-intervention group. It was projected that the men in the usual-care group would exhibit no important changes over the six-year-study period in blood-pressure and serum-cholesterol levels, and only minimal changes in smoking habits. The investigators predicted 442 deaths at the end of six years for men in the usual-care group.

But the actual findings, both in modification of risk factors and deaths, in the usual-care group were very different than anticipated. Deaths in the usual-care group were less than half those predicted. Sizable reductions had occurred in the levels of all three risk factors over the course of the study in the usual-care group. This was a surprising turn of events.

Clearly something dramatic was going on in the general population, as evidenced by the good showing in the usual-care control group—a group that was selected to resemble those people in the general population who stood a good chance of dying of heart disease.

As it turned out, many of the men in the usual-care group modified their own risk factors on the advice of their personal physicians or on their own. "The broad influence of health education in the United States aimed at modifying all the three risk factors" was another contributing element, according to the study investigators.

Although the risk factors declined less in the usual-care group than in the special-intervention group, the final data show no significant difference in the mortality of the men in the two groups after seven years. And what's more, mortality in both groups was lower than expected at the beginning of the clinical trial.

Efforts to modify risk factors were paying off in fewer deaths, and the MRFIT study confirms the success in reducing death rates from heart disease in this country, according to Edward N. Brandt, Jr., M.D., assistant secretary for health in the Department of Health and Human Services.

The study, Dr. Brandt said, again shows the value of reducing one's risks of coronary heart disease. The death rate for those who quit smoking, he said, even for one year, was about half that of those who did not quit. The lesson to be learned from the study is that middle-aged men may be able to reduce their risks of death from coronary heart disease by reducing high blood pressure, by lowering elevated cholesterol levels and by quitting smoking.

It is almost never too late. If you are aware of your risks and heed the specific guidelines presented in the chapters that follow, you may be doing something about your own destiny as well as the quality of your life.

4

THE CASE AGAINST CHOLESTEROL

In a secluded laboratory on the gray Gothic campus of the University of Chicago, the rich aroma of roast pork and simmering gravy bubbling with globules of fat wafted into the air. A band of rhesus monkeys—the same hearty variety in which the Rh factor of blood was discovered—clambered to attention. It was their way of sending compliments to the chef, Robert W. Wissler, M.D., who had designed this unique experiment and arranged for the unusual simian diet that included bacon and eggs, cheese, butter and cream.

Across the corridor an identical band of monkeys reacted equally enthusiastically to their fare of lean meats and less fat—the kind of diet recommended for humans by some health organizations and many nutritionists.

As Dr. Wissler had anticipated, fatty, cholesterol-laden patches developed in the coronary arteries of many in the "typical American diet" group, while most of those in the "prudent diet" group remained free of the disease.

Monkeys, it appeared, were just as susceptible to coronary artery disease as humans. But the experiment was far from finished. Dr. Wissler was determined to find out something much more important: Could the formation of plaques in the arteries be stopped by a reduction of the amount of cholesterol and saturated fat in the diet of the first group of monkeys? As the weeks and months passed, the emerging evidence was brighter than anyone had hoped. Not only did the prudent diet halt the disease, it had a cleansing effect on the coronary arteries themselves.

Since people cannot be tested in scientific experiments as rigidly controlled as those in monkeys, there is only presumptive evidence—some of it conflicting—that human coronary artery disease is related to diet. While it is clear that elevated levels of cholesterol in the blood constitute a risk, there is still much controversy over the role of dietary modification in preventing heart disease in man—and it may be that saturated fats and cholesterol in the diet are not of equal importance in all persons.

Strands of evidence in the complex web of data implicating blood cholesterol—as distinct from dietary cholesterol—with arterial disease date back at least as far as 1910, but knowledge about arterial disease associated with it goes back much further.

In 1755 Albrecht von Haller, a Swiss physician, revived a long-dormant Greek term to describe the softenings that occur on the inner walls of arteries. Because of their resemblance to gruel—a mush that peasants ate—he labeled the arterial softening *atheroma* (*ather* being the Greek word for gruel), and he noted that it often resulted in a stiff, hardened area in an artery.

The story does not pick up again until 1904, this time in France, with another physician who took his Swiss predecessor's concept to its logical conclusion, in the best of medical traditions, and coined the term *atherosclerosis.* In a definition that still stands today, he recognized that atherosclerosis is a type of arteriosclerosis—a type of hardening of the arteries. Its distinguishing characteristic is the presence of a greasy, crystalline substance that to Dr. von Haller looked like gruel. Six years later, in 1910, this substance was identified as cholesterol.

Atherosclerosis, then, is a cholesterol-laden scab that forms on the inner wall of an artery. It is thought to begin with some kind of damage in the delicate lining of an artery. Turbulence in the bloodstream from high blood pressure or an excess of the hormone epinephrine from stress has been suggested as a cause. Hormones in the damaged area stimulate the appearance of a natural Band-Aid, and a clot forms to cover the abrasion. But in the presence of elevated cholesterol in the blood, this natural self-healing process goes awry. Instead of slowly disintegrating, the clot may grow and be transformed into an atherosclerotic plaque with a core of cholesterol and cellular debris and with an exterior cap of calcium.

When such plaques finally enlarge to block the flow of blood through a coronary artery, or when one breaks loose and lodges downstream in a narrower section of the artery, the portion of the heart fed by this artery becomes starved for oxygen and is severely damaged. This sudden dramatic ending to a process that may have begun in adolescence, or even in childhood, is called a heart attack.

The details of this scenario did not become known overnight; they resulted from years of painstaking research. During the same time, parallel research into the risk factors for coronary artery disease and heart attack would narrow the field to a few leading suspects. From the beginning, cholesterol in the blood appeared to be one of them. But cholesterol is not *all* bad despite the fact that, in abnormal accumulations, it is a chief source of trouble within the arteries.

The human liver normally synthesizes about 1,000 mg (milligrams) of cholesterol a day from saturated fats in the diet, and cells utilize it as a basic ingredient in the assembly of normal male and female hormones, vitamin D, membranes for cells, and sheaths that protect nerve fibers, among other things. After the first six months of an individual's life, the liver's production of cholesterol is sufficient for all the body's needs. Nevertheless, the average American consumes about 600 mg of cholesterol a day from dietary sources such as eggs and meat. Saturated fats, which come chiefly from dairy products, animal fat and such oils as coconut and palm, can raise the level of cholesterol in the blood. It is only when there is an overabundance of cholesterol in the blood, or when a genetic deficiency impairs the body's ability to utilize cholesterol and fats, that problems apparently occur.

The association between diet and heart attacks first came to light incidentally in Europe during World War II. As food rations became short, with little meat, eggs, butter and milk, hospitals in various countries began reporting a curious trend. At St. Joseph's Hospital in Porsgrunn, Norway, the percentage of admissions for coronary heart disease fell by 50 percent. At the municipal hospitals in Rotterdam, Holland, there were only six heart-attack deaths in 1945—that country's leanest year. At hospitals in prisoner-of-war camps behind the Russian front, physicians reported little evidence of atherosclerosis.

But after the war, as affluence returned to Europe, so did heart attacks. By 1950, heart attacks in Rotterdam hospitals were back to the prewar rate. By 1954, the percentage of admissions for coronary heart disease at the hospital in Porsgrunn had climbed from 1.5 percent during the war years to 7 percent. And heart attacks among repatriated prisoners resumed with telling frequency as they returned to a high-fat diet.

The circumstantial evidence against excessive consumption of animal fats and cholesterol was becoming stronger, but more persuasive evidence awaited studies in the 1960s. The Seven Country Study, involving 12,000 people in Finland, Greece, Italy, Japan, the Netherlands, the United States and Yugoslavia, pinpointed the highest rates of coronary heart disease among those living in eastern Finland and in the United States, where diets high in animal fat predominated.

The men surveyed in Finland and the United States obtained 17 to 23 percent of their calories from saturated fats, largely in meat, eggs and dairy products. By contrast, populations with the lowest coronary-disease and death rates subsisted on low-fat diets, consisting principally of fish and inexpensive starches like rice, bread and potatoes.

The International Atherosclerosis Project discovered a significant relationship between cholesterol levels in the blood and severity of atherosclerosis in more than 31,000 people who died between 1960 and 1965 in fifteen cities throughout the world.

As significant as these studies were, they left one perplexing question unanswered: Was it genetic influences that accounted for the differences in serum (blood) cholesterol levels and coronary heart disease? To find the answer, researchers turned to certain populations of immigrants who, the theory went, carried native genes from a "low-fat" culture to a "high-fat" culture.

In the Ni-Hon-San Study, the blood cholesterol levels of native Japanese men (on low-fat diets) were appreciably lower than those of Japanese men who had moved to America and were on a typically American high-fat diet, and heart disease was reflected in this disparity, with a far lower rate among the men living in Japan.

It was similarly found that Yemenite Jews increased their cholesterol levels and rates of coronary heart disease when they emigrated to Israel and began to eat a "Western" diet. And the same effect was noted in a study of Neapolitans who had moved from Italy to Boston, when compared with another group that had remained in Naples.

Genes and heredity did not seem to be involved in a major way. In the late 1970s Kaare R. Norum, Ph.D., chairman of the Institute of Nutrition Research at the University of Oslo in Norway, sent questionnaires to 214 cardiologists, surgeons, pathologists and geneticists working in coronary research. Almost 99 percent saw a link between the amount of cholesterol in the blood and the development of coronary heart disease.

These sentiments were echoed by Jeremiah Stamler, M.D., chairman of the Department of Community Health and Preventive Medicine at Northwestern University Medical School and director of a research program there. Writing in the *Archives of Surgery*, Dr. Stamler characterized heart disease as an epidemic that is ravaging Western industrialized countries.

Yet, despite the extensive evidence, there is still a cholesterol controversy. A sizable number of physicians are not convinced that diet is directly related to heart disease. They point to the inescapable fact that there is no direct evidence that altering the diet can reduce heart disease. In general, they believe that most people in Western societies have "normal" levels of cholesterol and need not reduce their intake of it or of saturated fats.

The serum cholesterol level of the average American adult is about 225 mg in each 100 ml (milliliters) of serum. Levels up to 250 and sometimes even 300 have been considered acceptable. However, the University of Chicago's Dr. Wissler considers this range too high, and evidence from Framingham supports him. In an address to a medical symposium, he noted that "Ninety percent of the world's people, most of whom don't eat as we do, have levels of between 100 and 150 milligrams, and almost never die of coronary heart disease." He believes an ideal figure to aim for is 150 in adults.

But with few exceptions—among them vegetarians—people after age twenty-one in the United States rarely attain Dr. Wissler's ideal cholesterol level. Failure to do so, though, does not automatically mean heart disease. There is thought to be a healthy range. According to Frederick J. Stare, M.D., a former chairman of Harvard's Department of Nutrition, a good example of a safe cholesterol level is being set by "those of us in nutritional medicine who try to keep our own cholesterol in the range of 200 or lower."

When cholesterol is consistently above this level, there are various approaches to bring it down. Taking off excess weight is an obvious way, but it is not the only answer. Even a diet considered Spartan by most Americans will reduce the average person's level of cholesterol by only 10 to 15 percent—though many consider this to be a significant reduction. Exercising regularly and quitting cigarettes also help.

In the event that dietary restrictions and weight loss fail to bring down the cholesterol level, some physicians may prescribe a cholesterol-lowering drug, but none of the drugs available is wholly effective, and many have troublesome side effects.

One of the most confusing aspects of the cholesterol story is that some people with high levels never develop coronary heart disease, while others with moderate levels are stricken. This embarrassing flaw in the cholesterol theory of heart disease led Tavia Gordon of the National Institutes of Health to search through the institute's coronary heart disease records for a possible explanation.

It is a common experience of medical research that discoveries often come from places where they are least expected. Bacteria that led the way to the discovery of the cause of tuberculosis settled by sheer chance on a slice of potato in the office of an inquisitive country practitioner. Had Robert Koch, M.D., not noticed the strange growth on the remains of his previous day's lunch, he might not have isolated the tubercle bacillus and might never have won his Nobel Prize.

Tavia Gordon found what she was looking for: virtually all victims of coronary heart disease had disproportionately small amounts of high-density lipoprotein. She later found that people who were relatively free of the disease had high HDL levels.

HDLs occur as droplets in the bloodstream, where they transport excess cholesterol to the liver. Based on laboratory experiments, it was learned that HDL increased the rate at which cholesterol can be transported from cells.

The normal level of HDL in the blood apparently fluctuates with age and with the amount of cholesterol in the body. We are born with enough HDL to bind about 50 percent of our total serum cholesterol. As we grow older and eat the typical American diet, the ratio changes. The average American man has an HDL level that can bind only about 20 percent of his cholesterol; the average woman has an HDL level that can bind slightly more, about 25 percent. The difference, according to William Castelli, M.D., of the Framingham Study, may account for the lower incidence of coronary heart disease among women.

Other factors also seem to play a role in determining HDL levels. In a study on the hereditary aspects of HDL done by Charles J. Glueck, M.D., director of lipid and general clinical research at the University of Cincinnati Medical Center, families whose members regularly reached their eighties and nineties without serious heart disease were found to have HDL levels 50 percent and more above average. While the evidence is not as well documented, Stanford researchers found that long-distance runners have average HDL levels almost 50 percent above the level of people who do not engage in vigorous exercise. This finding suggests the possibility that the level of protective HDLs can be raised through medication or by some other process—or, conversely, that the level can be lowered by the way we live.

Researchers have found evidence for both circumstances. Alcohol in moderate amounts—a drink or two a day—appears to raise the HDL level. On the other hand, cigarette smoking seems to lower it. Fortunately, most things that *reduce* cholesterol also *increase* HDL.

While researchers continue to delve into the subplots of the cholesterol story, there is a nearly unbroken string of evidence, stretching back to the beginning of the century, that supports the original suspicion. Cholesterol in the blood is a major culprit—there is no longer any doubt about its relationship to heart disease.

5

THE DIET CONNECTION

Few murderers in history could match the ingenuity of Père Gourier, a wealthy landowner in postrevolutionary France whose unexpected and untraceable weapon was the gluttony of his prey. In the last decade of his life, it was Gourier's perverted hobby to select periodically a dining companion of limited means, to lavish upon him, day after day, the richest repasts and best wine, and then count the months until his victim dropped dead. Urged on by his host, himself a man of gargantuan appetite, the guest would literally gorge himself to an early grave. Eventually, reported Christian Guy in his *Illustrated History of French Cuisine*, Gourier succumbed during a steak-eating contest with one of his intended victims.

In one way or another, we are all at the mercy of the foods we consume. Hardly a day passes without a newspaper article warning of yet another hazardous food or an author promising miracles from the latest dietary fad. Amid the plethora of confusing information about what is healthy to eat and what is not, the question often heard is: "Whom can I trust?" Admittedly, the relationship between diet and health is frustratingly complex, and what works for one person may not work for another. But physicians, dieticians and nutrition researchers who have long been passionately interested in this subject have uncovered a few basic nutritional principles that apply to nearly everyone.

A diet lower in cholesterol and saturated fat may be better than one that is loaded with both these substances, and a diet (in this

The Fight Against Fat
What you should weigh

Suggested Weights for Heights

Persons with wide shoulders and hips and large wrists and ankles can consider themselves in the "large frame" category. Those with narrow shoulders and hips and small wrists and ankles can consider themselves as having a "small frame." Most people fall in the "medium frame" category. Your estimated ideal weight should not change as you become older.

Feet & Inches	Small Frame	Medium Frame	Large Frame
	lbs	lbs	lbs
5'3"	118	129	141
5'4"	122	133	145
5'5"	126	137	149
5'6"	130	142	155
5'7"	134	147	161
5'8"	139	151	166
5'9"	143	155	170
5'10"	147	159	174
5'11"	150	163	178
6'	154	167	183
6'1"	158	171	188
6'2"	162	175	192
6'3"	165	178	195

Feet & Inches	lbs	lbs	lbs
5'	100	109	118
5'1"	104	112	121
5'2"	107	115	125
5'3"	110	118	128
5'4"	113	122	132
5'5"	116	125	135
5'6"	120	129	139
5'7"	123	132	142
5'8"	126	136	146
5'9"	130	140	151
5'10"	133	144	156
5'11"	137	148	161
6'	141	152	166

Source: *The Healthy Approach to Slimming,* © American Medical Association.

case diet means an eating habit) that keeps you at your ideal weight is better for your heart than one that keeps you overweight. The key principle is moderation. There is no ideal diet, and none can guarantee health.

Gourier's bloated victims probably succumbed to a variety of disorders, not the least of which was heart disease. Partly because of data from the Framingham Study and others like it, physicians now know that it is not overeating itself that shortens life, but the conditions associated with it.

A steady diet of the wrong foods or excess weight from consistently eating too much have been implicated in diabetes, high blood pressure and excessive levels of cholesterol. Each of these conditions, in turn, has been found to increase the risk of heart attack. It is as if an internal conspiracy is launched at the lips and has repercussions throughout the body. Life-insurance actuarial statistics bear witness to this conspiracy. Over the decades that these statistics have been recorded, they have shown a steady increase in mortality with each extra pound of weight. This "extra" is the consequence of an imprudent diet, and it is the modern equivalent of Gourier's villainy.

In the current medical view, a little extra padding is not necessarily harmful. But a diet of high-caloric convenience foods and a lifestyle that is sedentary can push that "little extra" into the danger zone and put a continuous burden on the heart. As a general rule, ideal weight "is when your heart and lungs function well and your work performance is good," according to Maria Simonson, Ph.D., director of the Johns Hopkins University Health and Weight Program.

In more practical terms, height and weight tables, such as the one shown here, give the normal range for your age and sex. These figures are merely guidelines, though, and not hard-and-fast rules, as it is possible to be very overweight according to the chart, and still not be obese. The extra weight on a professional football player may well be muscle, not fat. Nursing mothers may be overweight as judged by the tables, but their extra pounds are necessary during breast-feeding, and those excess pounds tend to melt away with weaning.

To calculate your own ideal weight, it is a good idea to consult the charts and then put the figure you arrive at in perspective by taking the "pinch test." This is an at-home version of what many physicians concerned with weight reduction and physical conditioning do. By measuring the thickness of skinfolds, they can determine quite accurately the percentage of body fat. This should be between 5 and 15 percent of total weight for men, and 10 to 20 percent for women (who naturally have slightly more subcutaneous fat).

Using the at-home version, you can dispense with percentages. It is inches that count. Tense your left arm. If you can pinch more than an inch of skin at the back of your arm between your thumb and forefinger you are probably about 20 percent overweight and in the danger zone. Depending on your height, this could be ten, twenty or thirty pounds that, for the sake of your heart, you should not be carrying around. As a glance at the best-seller list quickly establishes, there are numerous ways advocated to lose those extra pounds, but the "battle of the bulge" must be won in the head before it can succeed at the stomach. Vanity aside, the heart will notice the difference it takes to shed those extra pounds even before the notches in the belt record the difference.

Research studies have demonstrated that the heart, in essence, breathes a sigh of relief as a person's weight declines to the ideal. It no longer has to pump blood through all that extra fat, nor must it strain so hard each time those extra pounds are carried up a flight of stairs. Furthermore, as the fat melts away, the blood's cholesterol level usually declines.

After assessing the effect of weight loss on the heart's function, physicians noticed that regardless of the number of different dietary approaches, the body knows only one way to lose weight: it must burn up more calories than it takes in as food. This formula underlies every successful diet. It is extraordinarily simple, and from a nutritionist's view, quite obvious. Yet most authors of books on how to lose weight do not say so, preferring instead to promote the latest fad. The fact is that there has never been an improvement on the basic formula, and unless the human body changes, there will not be any change in this single, effective way to lose weight. The essential message of any effective weight-loss diet can be condensed into a single sentence: in order to lose weight, you have to eat less or exercise more, preferably both.

Contrary to popular belief, tests at Harvard University have shown that exercise frequently suppresses the appetite rather than increasing it. In research there and at other centers, neurophysiologists have demonstrated that the appetite is regulated by a delicate mechanism in the hypothalamus, a small cluster of specialized cells at the base of the brain. This appetite regulator—"appestat," as it is called—monitors sugar, fat, protein and oxygen in the blood and reacts to chemical signals from the digestive system.

When we get enough exercise, the appestat balances caloric intake and outgo so precisely that many people do not vary more than a pound within a year. But when we fall into sedentary habits the appestat functions less effectively. It is then that we eat more than we should.

The type of exercise that strengthens the heart (discussed in the next chapter) will, according to the nutritionist Jean Mayer, Ph.D., D.Sc., not only burn off excess fat but also will reset the appestat so that it functions effectively. This process, though, is not entirely automatic. It can be helped along by adjustments in the type and amount of food that one consumes, and it is here, in this "help along" gray zone, that most diet books address themselves.

Unfortunately, the advice of most such books falls short of its promise. In the high-protein diet, for instance, the weight goes down because fluid is lost, not fat. This is because the kidneys require extra quantities of water from the body to flush away the nitrogen resulting from protein breakdown. Not only is this diet ineffective in shrinking the fat globules of adipose tissue, but its effect lasts only until the next few bottles of soda or glasses of water are thirstily quaffed. Low-carbohydrate diets also appear to work at first, but they fail for the same reason—a temporary loss of water, not fat.

In a critical review of the popular "revolutionary" diets and similar low-carbohydrate regimens, the American Medical Association's Council on Foods and Nutrition warned that the risk of coronary artery disease may inadvertently be escalated by any diet that advocates an "unlimited" intake of saturated fats and cholesterol-rich foods.

The central tenet of a successful dietary regimen is to eat a variety of foods in moderation. If you know you have a high cholesterol level, you should seek dietary advice from your physician. Even if your serum cholesterol level is not elevated, you should still moderate your fat intake. This may be accomplished with the help of the nutritional information provided on food labels. Since levels of blood cholesterol do not necessarily reflect dietary practices, there is usually no need to restrict yourself or your family to an extremely low cholesterol diet unless your physician has specifically advised it.

The idea of producing low-cholesterol foods began over a crock of Boston baked beans. As Helen B. Brown, Ph.D., a leading nutritionist at the Cleveland Clinic, recalls, "Members of the clinic's research division were coming for supper, and I had prepared a large earthenware pot of beans with beer, mustard, molasses and salt pork, following a good old New England recipe."

No one at the supper party expected that people would happily switch to a liquid formula, but they wondered aloud about designing solid foods around the low-cholesterol concept. From this humble beginning, in 1957, Dr. Brown pioneered the development of such new foods as soft polyunsaturated margarine. Collaborating with other food scientists and food manufacturers, she was instrumental in devising some ninety special food products that were made available to hundreds of people in the National Comparative Diet and Heart Study. The two-year experiment succeeded in taste appeal and in lowering cholesterol levels in people whose blood cholesterol had been elevated, and its legacy is evident on supermarket and grocery shelves around the country.

Fats in the diet are essential for normal growth, healthy skin and the transportation of vitamins to the tissues; we cannot do without them. People who do not have high cholesterol levels and are free of other coronary risk factors have no need to curtail saturated fats or cholesterol in the food they eat. Again, moderation, and not elimination, is the chief cautionary note. Following are some common questions concerning diet answered by Dr. Brown:

What are the differences in the various types of meat?
Meat is high in protein, essential for building muscles and maintaining other body tissues. But it is also almost always rich in fat. A 6-ounce fried hamburger, for example, contains about six teaspoons of liquid fat, while a 6-ounce portion of fat-trimmed round steak contains only about two teaspoons of liquid fat.

Liver, like other organ meats, is very high in cholesterol, but it is an important source of iron and other valuable nutrients. Fish is lower in fat and has more polyunsaturates than meat. Shellfish is also low in fat, but shrimp is high in cholesterol. With the exception of duck and goose, poultry is a lean source of protein.

What is the latest word on eggs?

Egg yolks have been singled out as one of the leading dietary sources of cholesterol. However, eggs are also a good source of protein. For healthy people with no cholesterol problem, a limited number of eggs can be part of a sound nutritional diet. But like other foods, they should be consumed in moderation and along with a variety of other staples, including vegetables, fruits, cereals and breads.

What about other dairy products such as milk and cheese?

Soft cheeses, such as hoop, farmer's, mozzarella, and sapsago, have much less fat than the hard varieties. So if you are watching your diet, or if you have to lower your cholesterol, you may want to rely on soft cheeses and low-fat milk rather than those with a higher fat content. Otherwise, if you are not having any problems with your cholesterol level, enjoy yourself. As the Food and Nutrition Board of the National Academy of Sciences concluded in May 1980, "good food that provides appropriate proportions of nutrients should not be regarded as a poison, a medicine, or a talisman. It should be eaten and enjoyed."

What about the great American dessert—ice cream?

It has an average butterfat content of 10 to 20 percent, and it is an occasional (not daily) treat that need not be eliminated from the American table unless your doctor's dietary advice says so.

Except for butter, aren't all spreads and oils really alike?

This is a very tricky and confusing area for the average shopper. A tablespoon of butter contains 35 mg of cholesterol. Some "no cholesterol" hydrogenated hard margarines contain coconut or palm oil that has as much saturated fat as butter. If you are following your doctor's recommendations for a low-cholesterol, low-fat diet, it is important to read the labels for nutritional information and keep on reading them because the mixtures of fats may change as prices change. Look for the P/S (polyunsaturated/saturated) fat ratio, or if it is not listed, the total grams of polyunsaturated and

saturated fats per tablespoon. From these figures, you can determine the ratio yourself. Any ratio of 1/1 is good, but 2/1 is better.

For the purpose of figuring out their influence on cholesterol,
fats are classified into three groups. The *saturated* variety, found
in meats, cream and such vegetable oil as coconut and palm, can
temporarily elevate cholesterol in the blood. The *monosaturated*
fats, found in olive and peanut oil, have little or no effect on blood
cholesterol. The *polyunsaturated* fats, found in corn, sunflower
and safflower oil, tend to reduce cholesterol in the blood.

So, again, check the label whenever you buy oil, shortening or
margarine for the P/S ratio, and note whether the vegetable oils
have been hydrogenated—that is, converted to be as harmful as
cholesterol.

What else is necessary for a balanced diet?

Citrus fruit, berries, melon, broccoli or tomatoes are all good
sources of vitamins, particularly vitamin C. Carbohydrates and
starch from such foods as pasta, whole-grain bread and cereals, and
even potatoes, are far less fattening than commonly believed and
provide vitamins and fiber necessary for good digestion.

Starch has an undeserved reputation for adding fat to the body.
In reality, most starchy foods are rather low in calories. A medi-
um-sized baked potato, for instance, has 90 calories—about the
same number as a ripe banana or an apple. It is only when that
potato is garnished with sour cream or dripping with a fatty spread
that its caloric content soars.

Is it possible to dine out and still stick to a sane diet?

One prominent heart-disease researcher calls it virtually impossible, particularly if you are tempted by mouth-watering descriptions. But you can stay within your physician's prescribed caloric,
cholesterol and fat limits if you order broiled meat or fish—cooked
without butter and served without rich sauces—or poultry, or
salads with polyunsaturated dressing.

Veal and pasta dishes, if they are not made with cream or cheese,
are moderately low in cholesterol, as is most Chinese food. One
cautionary note, though: Anyone with a tendency toward high
blood pressure should be aware that soy sauce and monosodium
glutamate, which are used plentifully in most Chinese restaurants,
have a high sodium content. (See pages 72 and 150 for more on salt.)

Should fast-food meals be avoided?

Again, the happy answer is "no." Even pizza is fine, but not as a steady diet. The same goes for those quick burgers. Edwin Traisman, the program administrator of the Food Research Institute at the University of Wisconsin, has calculated the effect on an average man who eats all three meals at a fast-food hamburger chain, something even the corporate executives of the firm do not suggest. The total cholesterol content comes to 302 mg, a modest amount. The caloric value added up to 2,632, again a moderate number for an active man. Fat intake equals 1,058 calories, or 40 percent of the total—about the national daily average.

Some fast-food hamburgers are relatively lean, says Traisman. The meat contains no more than 20 percent fat, versus 30 percent in standard retail hamburger meat. The milkshakes are made with iced milk, which contains only 2.9 to 3.1 percent fat. The French fries, cooked in a mixture of cottonseed oil and beef fat contain 15.3 percent fat. These are typical percentages in the fast-food industry.

Fast-food calorie count

	Hamburger Chain #1		Hamburger Chain #2		Chicken		Pizza		Taco	
	Item	Calories	Item	Calories	Item	Calories	Item	Calories	Item	Calories
Typical Meal	Two-patty hamburger	541	Superburger	606	Chicken Dinner* (extra crispy)	950	Thick Deluxe**	640	Taco	186
	Fries	211	Fries	214					Beef burrito	466
	Cola (8 oz.)	96	Cola (8 oz.)	96	Cola (8 oz.)	96	Cola (8 oz.)	96	Cola (8 oz.)	96
		848		916		1046		736		748
Other Items	Quarter-pound cheeseburger	518	Cheeseburger	305	Chicken Dinner*	830	Thick w/pepperoni	560	Tostada	179
	Fish sandwich	402	Hamburger	252	Drumstick	136	Thin Deluxe	510	Burrito Deluxe	457
	Quarter-pound hamburger	418	Vanilla shake	332	Wing	151	Thin w/pepperoni	430		

*Chicken dinner includes mashed potatoes, gravy, cole slaw, roll, and three pieces of chicken.
**Based on serving of one-half 10-inch pizza.
Source: Ross Laboratories (Perspectives on Fast Foods. Dietetic Currents)

Fortunately, it is not necessary to have a degree in nutrition to plan a well-balanced diet. "The important thing to remember," says Dr. Brown, "is that no one food does everything. But most foods have something to offer." If you choose a variety of foods, eat moderate portions and hold sweets and extras to a minimum, you will not need to count calories or worry about fat percentages. If you succeed in following these simple rules, you will learn the joys and reap the benefits of a slim and, we hope, healthy body.

The Fight Against Fat
Counting your calories . . .

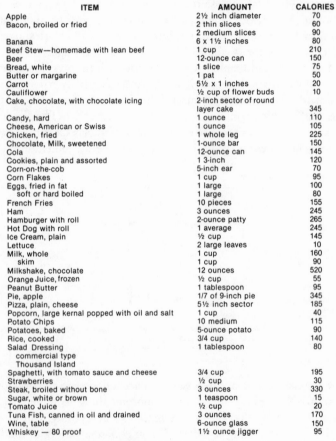

ITEM	AMOUNT	CALORIES
Apple	2½ inch diameter	70
Bacon, broiled or fried	2 thin slices	60
	2 medium slices	90
Banana	6 x 1½ inches	80
Beef Stew—homemade with lean beef	1 cup	210
Beer	12-ounce can	150
Bread, white	1 slice	75
Butter or margarine	1 pat	50
Carrot	5½ x 1 inches	20
Cauliflower	½ cup of flower buds	10
Cake, chocolate, with chocolate icing	2-inch sector of round layer cake	345
Candy, hard	1 ounce	110
Cheese, American or Swiss	1 ounce	105
Chicken, fried	1 whole leg	225
Chocolate, Milk, sweetened	1-ounce bar	150
Cola	12-ounce can	145
Cookies, plain and assorted	1 3-inch	120
Corn-on-the-cob	5-inch ear	70
Corn Flakes	1 cup	95
Eggs, fried in fat	1 large	100
soft or hard boiled	1 large	80
French Fries	10 pieces	155
Ham	3 ounces	245
Hamburger with roll	2-ounce patty	265
Hot Dog with roll	1 average	245
Ice Cream, plain	½ cup	145
Lettuce	2 large leaves	10
Milk, whole	1 cup	160
skim	1 cup	90
Milkshake, chocolate	12 ounces	520
Orange Juice, frozen	½ cup	55
Peanut Butter	1 tablespoon	95
Pie, apple	1/7 of 9-inch pie	345
Pizza, plain, cheese	5½ inch sector	185
Popcorn, large kernal popped with oil and salt	1 cup	40
Potato Chips	10 medium	115
Potatoes, baked	5-ounce potato	90
Rice, cooked	3/4 cup	140
Salad Dressing commercial type Thousand Island	1 tablespoon	80
Spaghetti, with tomato sauce and cheese	3/4 cup	195
Strawberries	½ cup	30
Steak, broiled without bone	3 ounces	330
Sugar, white or brown	1 teaspoon	15
Tomato Juice	½ cup	20
Tuna Fish, canned in oil and drained	3 ounces	170
Wine, table	6-ounce glass	150
Whiskey — 80 proof	1½ ounce jigger	95

Source: Home and Garden Bulletin No. 153, U.S. Dept. of Agriculture, Prepared by Consumer Food Economics Research Division.

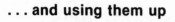

. . . and using them up

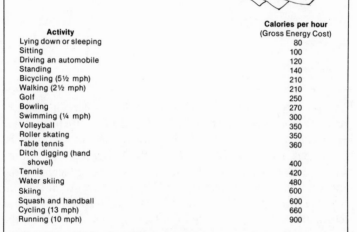

Activity	Calories per hour (Gross Energy Cost)
Lying down or sleeping	80
Sitting	100
Driving an automobile	120
Standing	140
Bicycling (5½ mph)	210
Walking (2½ mph)	210
Golf	250
Bowling	270
Swimming (¼ mph)	300
Volleyball	350
Roller skating	350
Table tennis	360
Ditch digging (hand shovel)	400
Tennis	420
Water skiing	480
Skiing	600
Squash and handball	600
Cycling (13 mph)	660
Running (10 mph)	900

Source: *Basic Bodywork for Fitness and Health,* Published by the American Medical Association.

6

THE BENEFITS
OF EXERCISE

High on a steep hill in the Liechtenstein Alps, a certain multilingual innkeeper is reputed to have developed a sure-fire formula for identifying the nationality of his guests. The inn can only be reached via a steep, serpentine footpath. At the top, before they have a chance to say a word, visitors are warmly greeted by the innkeeper in their native tongue. When asked how he accomplishes this Sherlock Holmesian feat, the host explains in a most elementary fashion: "I can tell the Germans by their shoes, the Swedes by their blond hair, the French by their clothes, and the Americans because they are out of breath."

The cardiologist who tells this story is not amused by it. To Ira J. Bernstein, M.D., of Highland Park, Illinois, it illustrates the point that despite the physical-fitness "craze," countless numbers of Americans are dangerously out of shape. They do not exercise, and their hearts and bodies are not strong enough to meet anything but minimum demands.

The heart is a muscle, and like other muscles, it performs a measurable quantity of work each time it contracts. The amount of work is reflected by the amount of blood the heart is able to pump with each beat. The average heart pumps 2 to 2 1/2 ounces of blood in less than a second; then it rests for an instant and pumps again. This cycle of work-rest-work-rest is repeated not hundreds of times a day, not thousands of times a day, but at the very minimum a hundred thousand times a day, and thus the work the heart performs takes on awesome dimensions.

During an average day, when the heart is neither called on to do much extra work nor overly taxed by anxiety or stress, it pumps over 2,000 gallons of blood, at the rate of 6 quarts a minute, through 60,000 miles of blood vessels, keeping 75 trillion cells nourished with vital oxygen. It has been estimated that the daily work of the human heart in propelling blood is equivalent to lifting 124 tons to a height of one foot. And the heart does this routinely, resting only a fraction of a second between beats. No other organ works so hard to meet the body's basic demands.

For the heart, this is the minimum level of performance, ground zero. But again like other muscles, it has reserves. In an emergency, or during strenuous exercise, the heart can more than triple its pumping rate in a matter of seconds, and its output may climb as high as 36 quarts a minute. These peaks, though, can be attained only for short times unless the heart has been strengthened and its reserves extended by exercise.

You do not have to be a fanatic about exercise nor a sprinter nor a construction worker to reap the benefits of a strengthened heart. The crucial conclusion from hundreds of studies on athletes, manual laborers and sedentary workers is that a stronger heart—a heart that can tap its reserves without exhausting consequences—is often a healthier heart.

After recording the normal heart rate of thousands of people, cardiologists initially noticed an enormous range, both higher and lower than the average 72 beats per minute. People in good physical condition, whose hearts had been strengthened by the activity of their work or through conscientious exercise, had a lower resting heart rate than people who had engaged in little or no physical activity.

Surprisingly, the "normal" heart rate for the best-conditioned athletes was so slow—in the 40-beat-per-minute or lower range—that many cardiologists once considered the enlarged, sluggish athletic heart to be an abnormality. Now it is known that having a normally slow heart rate does not jeopardize the heart's capacity. In fact, the strengthened athletic heart pumps out more blood on the average beat than a less fit, less well-conditioned heart. Thus, it can beat at a slower pace and still meet the body's requirements.

The fit heart not only idles at a lower speed—measured by taking the pulse—but does not have to strain during peak activity. It can accelerate to a higher rate and stay there longer than the unexercised heart when great demands are put upon it. For practical purposes, this means that a well-conditioned person can shovel snow, for example, or push a car, or run to catch a bus without overburdening his heart.

More important, though, having a slow heart rate can be a distinct advantage in terms of cardiac health. Jeremiah Stamler, M.D., of Northwestern University Medical School, and his colleagues found that men with resting heart rates of 60 beats a minute or slower had two to three times less chance of dying from coronary heart disease as did men whose heart rates were above 80 at rest. The slower pulse rate of a well-conditioned person is a reflection of a strong heart, and a strong heart presumably is less susceptible to damage from stress and strain.

Before mechanization and automation, many people received the benefits of a good measure of healthful exercise—stronger hearts and slower pulses—from the labor they did to earn a living, and this was reflected in heart-disease statistics. A Purdue University study of brothers revealed that those who stayed on their Indiana farms had healthier hearts and fewer heart attacks than did their siblings who moved to the city for less physically taxing jobs behind desks.

The same pattern is apparent in an English study, done in 1953, which showed that fatal heart attacks were twice as prevalent among clerks as among letter carriers, and in an Israeli study, conducted a decade later, which concluded with similar statistics for clerks and field workers.

Herman K. Hellerstein, M.D., of Case Western Reserve University, who has analyzed the work expended in scores of occupations, has found that even fewer of us nowadays can depend upon our jobs to keep us in condition. Housework, though, still ranks high on the calorie-burning scale. In fact, Dr. Hellerstein has discovered that it takes more energy to clean house, for example, than it does to work in most factories.

Many people believe that they are more active on the job than they actually are. They fail to realize that the fatigue is from emotional stress, not from physical activity. At best, most people use only 20 percent of their maximum energy capacity on the job. Clearly, this is not enough to keep the heart in tip-top condition. So—do you have to change your occupation to ditchdigging or run marathons to have a healthier heart? The encouraging answer is that you do not have to do either, or anything else that drastic.

Until a few years ago, it was generally believed that all you had to do to strengthen your heart was to exercise until you were short of breath, perspiring and feeling an undefined but pleasant sense of fatigue. But after numerous studies on specific exercise regimens, that vague prescription has been substantially refined into a medically sound heart exercise plan.

In England, a study of nearly 9,000 government workers, aged forty to fifty-four, showed that those who walked twenty minutes or more a day on their way to or from work had only two-thirds as many abnormal electrocardiograms (indicating heart damage) as those who did not walk at all.

Strenuous leisure-time exercise appears to be even better for the heart. In a study of 17,000 Harvard alumni, the University of California's Ralph S. Paffenberger, Jr., M.D., found strong statistical evidence that an individual's heart-attack risk diminishes if he engages in such strenuous sports as swimming, running, basketball, handball, squash or tennis. Casual sports such as golf, bowling or baseball do not seem to help. The study also showed that *total* overall activity on and off the job was important. "Heart-attack rates declined with increasing activity," Dr. Paffenberger said, "whether measured as stairs climbed, blocks walked, or strenuous sports."

Cardiologists and exercise physiologists have devised a simple formula, based on these and other studies, that determines almost to the minute and pulse beat how much exercise is best for your heart. It is a formula that can be personalized to your specifications, depending on your age, your present level of physical conditioning, and your cardiac health.

For most people whose hearts are sound to begin with, this means only about twenty minutes of all-out exercise every other day. The key principle, though—and the concept that makes this plan different from all the others—is that in order for the exercise to be beneficial, it must be just strenuous enough to push your pulse rate into your own "target zone," which is between 70 and 85 percent of your maximum attainable heart rate (220, minus your age).

Thus, if you are fifty years old, subtract 50 from 220 to get your maximum heart rate—170. Then multiply this figure by .70 and by .85 to calculate the target zone—a pulse rate of 119 to 144. If you are thirty years old, subtract 30 from 220 to get your maximum heart rate—190. Then multiply this by .70 and by .85 for your personalized target zone—133 to 161.

The principle of this prescription is that the heart is a muscle and must be exercised *above* a certain level to increase its strength. To get into the target zone and stay there, you must learn to take your pulse frequently. When you are exercising strenuously, your heart pounds and the pulse is strong and easily located by placing your fingertips on either side in front of the ear or on the wrist. Stop the exercise momentarily, and immediately count your pulse for ten seconds; then multiply by six to get the count for one minute (do not count longer, the pulse rate rapidly drops off). Then resume exercising.

After doing this a number of times, you will be able to sense by the feel of your rapid heartbeat when you are in the target zone, and you will not need to take your pulse as often. Exercise in the target zone forces the heart to work hard pumping blood to other active muscles throughout the body, but not so hard that it is unduly strained. It leaves an important cardiac cushion above the target zone, so you can be assured that you are exercising in a safe yet heart-strengthening range.

If you are very sedentary, over thirty-five, or have ever been told you have a heart condition, you should undergo an exercise stress test in a physician's office or in a hospital's cardiology department before starting a strenuous exercise program. You must be well-rested and prepared to sweat and strain on the day you take your stress test, for the idea is to tax your body machine to the limit. The exercise begins easily but becomes tougher every one to three minutes until finally, five, ten or twenty minutes later, you have reached your maximum exertion. This is the point at which the heart cannot beat any faster and is unable to deliver any more oxygen to the tissues.

Your exercise prescription will be based upon this peak of your heart's endurance. If you attained a heart rate of 172 beats per minute, for example, your 70 to 85 percent target zone will be 120 to 145. In some exercise programs the physician will recommend the exact number of yards to run or laps to swim, or whatever, in the weeks ahead. In others, the choice and length of exercise will be left to you, provided you keep within safe target-zone limits.

As the heart strengthens through weeks and months of exercise, it apparently undergoes other beneficial changes as well. Certain studies indicate that vigorous exercise actually may stimulate the growth of extra capillaries which branch off small coronary vessels to feed the heart—and this may provide an extra measure of safety against heart attack. Like other muscles in the body, the heart muscle increases in bulk with exercise. Although the actual number of muscle cells does not change, the muscle fibers increase in size, and additional oxygen is required to supply the cells' increased capacity. This anatomical change is paralleled by physiological mechanisms within cells which may cause the release of certain chemical factors that stimulate capillary growth. (Similar cellular activities take place, for example, during the healing process when the skin and underlying tissue is cut.) Known as the collateral circulation, these extra vessels can, in practical terms, not only provide the heart muscle with more blood but also reroute the flow around obstructed portions of the larger coronary arteries, bypassing atherosclerotic clogs or blood clots.

Exercise may also help prevent heart attacks by increasing the diameter of the main coronary arteries, enabling them, in theory, to carry a sufficient supply of blood to the heart, even though the vessels themselves may be crusty with plaques. Not all types of exercise, however, strengthen the heart. Lifting weights and performing calisthenics may build muscles, loosen joints, and promote flexibility, but neither exercise lasts long enough, nor is strenuous enough to coax the heart rate into the target zone.

In the view of many cardiologists, the two best heart-strengthening exercises are jogging and swimming. But brisk walking, cycling and fast-paced ball games—for instance, squash or handball—demand enough sustained effort to expand lung capacity, dilate blood vessels and get the heart beating in the target zone.

Since boredom and inconvenience are the twin enemies of fitness, no one can dictate what type of exercise will suit you the best. The only recommendation is: Choose the type—or mixture —of activity that you can build into your life, just as you build in time to take a daily shower or brush your teeth.

The experience of a professor at the University of California in San Diego proves the wisdom of this advice. Upon recovering from a heart attack, which he suffered at age forty-nine, he tried one elaborate exercise program after another. They all fell by the wayside because he found them too time-consuming. Finally the chairman of the university's physical education department convinced him to accept a substitute plan: whenever the professor had to visit the washroom, he would use a facility on a lower floor, taking the stairs both ways. Eventually he was taking a break every hour to walk from his fifth-floor laboratory down to the first-floor washroom and back again—just for the exercise! The extra activity made him feel so good that he actually did more work in less time and, on his own, began jogging every morning with his dog.

Others, of course, have found different ways to add exercise to their lives, and so can you. Sell your riding lawnmower. Get rid of the upstairs phone that saves you extra steps. Ride a bicycle or walk to your commuting station. If you must drive, park your car half a mile from work and run the rest of the way. Jog in place while watching the morning news.

If you exercise within your target zone for twenty to thirty minutes a day, three times a week, you should begin noticing an improvement in your cardiovascular performance within a month. You will be able to run more miles or swim more laps—and you can probably keep improving week after week.

The first informal rule of an exercise program is: start slow and take it easy. If you plan to jog, try only short distances at first, and alternate jogging with walking. This will not only get your heart and lungs used to the new routine but also minimize muscle aches and pains. Do not exercise—or use extreme caution—when you are not feeling well, when you are overtired or when it is very hot or cold. And stop *immediately* if you have any chest pain or feel dizzy, and notify your doctor.

A good technique borrowed from the athletic field is to begin every exercise gingerly, with a warm-up of five to ten minutes, which prevents sudden taxing of the heart and circulation. It's not a good idea, for example, to start your morning run the moment you step out the front door. Walk or alternately walk and jog for a couple of blocks until your body gets used to the idea.

Similarly, following strenuous exercise, taper off with a five- to ten-minute cool-down. If you have been running, walk for a while, as athletes do at the end of a race. If you stop abruptly, you may trap too much blood in the muscles of the lower portion of your body. Then not enough blood circulates back toward the brain and heart, and you may experience dizziness, nausea or even extra heartbeats. (Such heart palpitations should alert you to call your doctor.)

One of the most difficult concepts for people to grasp, according to Dolores Doehler, who is health and fitness director at the Northwest Suburban YMCA in Des Plaines, Illinois, is that exercise will not wear them out. "We tell them that they're going to be somewhat tired right after exercise," she said, "but in the long run they will feel better and have *more energy.*" In physiological terms, when the heart's output is increased, the fatigue level drops.

Noel D. Nequin, M.D., a runner himself, and director of a leading cardiac rehabilitation program at Chicago's Swedish Covenant Hospital, puts the prevailing medical view on exercise and the heart this way: "Exercise is important as a take-off point toward a new lifestyle aimed at reducing the risk factors for heart disease. It helps reduce blood pressure. It helps reduce obesity. It improves fitness, work capacity and endurance. It eases tension and improves psychological well-being and, at the same time, exercise makes it easier to quit smoking and change your diet." Hundreds of physicians and thousands of people in other walks of life are proving these points every day.

It simply makes all the sense in the world to get out there and exercise.

7

STRESS

To the untrained eye, the waiting room in the San Francisco suite shared by two private practitioners bears all the usual evidence of a well-trafficked doctor's office. A pile of once neatly stacked magazines lies in a clutter across the top of a side table. Heavy, anxious footsteps have worn deeply into the nap of the carpet. Fingermark smudges mar the luster of the wooden armchairs and sofa cushions sag under the accumulation of the troubled weight they were meant to support. Nothing out of the ordinary, or so the two doctors thought until they were visited by an upholsterer who mentioned the curious fact that the signs of wear were only on the *front edges* of the cushions and seats.

It would have been an inconsequential observation in any other office. But the doctors here—both perceptive specialists—grasped the importance of the remark immediately. Their patients, at least many of them, cannot sit still. They fidget on the front of the chairs, probably glancing at their watches every few seconds. They are time-conscious—pent up with the feeling that they have to accomplish something and not sit idly as the world rushes by.

The worn front edges of the cushions are just another indication that these people are on edge, so to speak, all the time, striving against the constraints of time and limits of their own endurance. They are also victims of heart disease, and that is what brought them to the waiting room of the two cardiologists, Meyer Friedman, M.D., and Ray H. Rosenman, M.D.

Drs. Friedman and Rosenman began noticing that most of their patients who had developed premature heart disease—that is, heart disease before age sixty-five—were aggressive, competitive personality types. To find out if other physicians noticed the same trend, they initially surveyed one hundred internists. The answers matched their own. Even a group of San Francisco businessmen identified "excessive competitive drive and meeting deadlines" as the outstanding characteristics of friends who had suffered heart attacks.

The closer the two cardiologists looked, the clearer the pattern became. Among the hundreds of men and women they talked to and examined, they found seven times as much coronary heart disease in the frazzled and harried subjects as in their slower-paced, more relaxed counterparts. In the best-selling book based on their research, *Type A Behavior and Your Heart,* Drs. Friedman and Rosenman conclude that a person with a hard-driving, time-conscious personality—whom they have labeled Type A—seems to be more susceptible to heart attack than does the placid, easygoing Type B.

Their findings were confirmed first at Columbia University's College of Physicians and Surgeons, where cardiologists detected severely narrowed coronary arteries in 82 percent of the patients with suspected heart disease who had previously been classified as Type A, and again in the Framingham Study, where researchers, after an eight-year study, found that Type As were at least twice as likely as Type Bs to develop angina, a heart attack or coronary heart disease. Office work proved especially hazardous for Type As. Fully 26.4 percent of Type A men aged forty-five to fifty-four in white-collar jobs developed coronary heart disease during the eight-year period, as compared with only 9.1 percent of white-collar Type Bs. Type A women faired little better, developing more than three times as much angina and twice as much coronary heart disease as did the Type B women in the study.

On the basis of their own extensive research, Friedman and Rosenman are convinced that Type A people actually seek out a hectic environment that puts undue stress upon them. Then they customarily overreact to the stress and out of proportion to the importance of whatever provoked them. The result is, the two cardiologists say, that Type As flare up easily, and their lives are filled with one emotional upheaval after another.

Type A people often walk and talk rapidly. They're likely to finish your sentences for you if you dawdle. They are usually the first to sound their horns in a traffic jam. They may stew while waiting five minutes for a table in a restaurant, then eat so quickly that they barely taste their food. Leisure often makes them feel vaguely guilty. Relaxation is anathema. Their lives, psychologists who have probed them say, are a struggle against time, toward achievement and recognition. They are, in effect, cauldrons of stress.

Most of us are a mix of types A and B. Sometimes, when life's situation is complex, we become too much "A," but we fall back into "B" and ease along. At some point, we are all "stressed."

Stress. The word alone is resonant with meaning. It is a rubber band stretched to the breaking point. It is the phone ringing and the baby crying and the roast burning. It is a poor grade, a missed opportunity, a glowing oil-pressure light on the dashboard of your car.

It can be everywhere or nowhere in particular. It can be vague or certain. We have an endless stream of aphorisms to describe it. The molehill that becomes a mountain. The eggs that don't hatch into chickens. The bridges that are crossed before you get to them. The worm that slowly turns. The wart that grows with worry.

The concept of stress is so ingrained in our language that, as Paul J. Rosch, M.D., of the American Institute of Stress has pointed out, it is hard to believe that it was medically defined only thirty years ago by Hans Selye, M.D., Ph.D., D.Sc., a brilliant medical researcher then at the University of Montreal who borrowed the word from physics. To Selye's way of thinking, stress is an individual's response to a traffic jam or an infection or a deadline. In other words, it is not the situation itself, but the reaction to the situation that causes the stress. In the Selye formula, anything that evokes emotions, such as a traffic jam or a note from the boss, is a stressor. But in everyday parlance, Selye's strict terminology did not catch on. His concept, though—that an ill-chosen word, a mindless error or a forgotten step can produce disease—did make a lasting impression on physicians and laymen alike.

Even so, the definition and measurement of stress continues to elude medical science in much the same way that the discovery of bacteria eluded scientists before the discovery of the microscope. They knew something was causing infections, and some of them went as far as to predict the existence of bacteria, but until they could see the minute culprits, they had no definitive evidence. This is the frustrating position some researchers find themselves in today with regard to stress. From laboratory experiments they know "it" causes harm. But how much "it" is bad? And what can be done to ward "it" off?

As late as 1979, the deceptively simple questions still lacked answers. Writing about stress in the *Journal of the American Medical Association* that year, Dr. Rosch claimed that "we all know what it is and, at the same time, nobody knows what it really is except that it is obviously different things for different people." That is as good a definition as any.

Stress may come in different shapes, forms and sizes, but the human body responds to it in a single, time-honored way that has remained essentially unaltered since prehistoric times, when our ancestral Homo sapiens had to survive tooth and nail in the real jungle.

Times may have changed, but anger, fear and anxiety still create the same complicated defensive reaction—sometimes known as the fight or flight syndrome—within our bodies as they did in the original Homo sapiens. Whether the threat is mental or physical, signals from the hypothalamus—the internal drummer at the base of the brain—trigger the release of adrenalin, which girds the body for action. At the urging of this powerful hormone, the heart strengthens and quickens its beat, echoing against the eardrums in an audible pounding as additional blood is rushed to the muscles and brain. The blood pressure rises. The liver empties fuel, fatty acids and cholesterol into the veins. The blood itself becomes stickier—better able to clot in the event of a wound in the forthcoming fight or flight.

In nature, as in sports or strenuous exercise, the violent muscular movements accompanying the fight or flight would use up the excess hormones, sugar, fat and cholesterol. But the civilized Type A is stymied. All day long, as worrysome encounter follows another, the undissipated stress chemicals continue to bathe the tissues, squeezing extra cholesterol into the blood and raising the blood pressure to the point where tiny rips may occur in the arterial walls. Blood flowing over these tiny rips develops small eddies, or disruptions in the current, like a stream flowing around a rock. Clots can form in these areas, and this could be the beginning of an atherosclerotic plaque. Through this combination, Drs. Friedman and Rosenman believe, stress causes the coronary damage that can result in a heart attack.

For a long time many people, physicians included, found it difficult to accept the idea that physical damage, such as heart disease, could result from continual mental stress. Convincing evidence, though, began pouring out of laboratories in the 1960s and 1970s. Animals could be afflicted with a variety of ailments, from accelerated atherosclerosis to heart attacks, by being exposed to stress. Then, in a series of forthright psychological tests devised to frustrate and aggravate but not physically harm the human subject, a startling blood-pressure finding came to light. The physiologists who administered the deceptively difficult mathematical part of the oral quiz, while measuring heart rate and blood pressure, discovered that emotional stress puts a greater strain on the heart than physical stress.

During physical stress from vigorous exercise they found that the diastolic, or lower, figure of the blood-pressure reading customarily drops, indicating that arteries throughout the body are expanding healthily to ease the flow of blood to all tissues. But during emotional stress the diastolic pressure goes up as the body tenses, putting additional strain on the heart.

According to Drs. Friedman and Rosenman, Type A people are particularly susceptible to the wear and tear of stress for the simple reason that they expose themselves to a continuous stream of stress in everything they do. They almost always set deadlines or quotas for themselves at home and at work, whereas Type Bs do this only occasionally. Type As carry the troubles of the office with them wherever they go. Type Bs are able to relax away from their desks, and rarely, if ever, bring work home.

Because these behavioral patterns are usually established in childhood, it may be difficult, but not impossible, for a Type A person to change. Dr. Friedman himself has had a coronary. He says he was once a Type A, and he is guiding himself into being a Type B. Thus, the inventor of the terms thinks one can modify the type by a sustained effort to change lifestyle and stress response. But Type A does not have to change altogether. The emphasis, according to one chairman who frequently leads symposiums on stress, should be on coping with stressful situations.

Charles Swencionis, Ph.D., who made that pronouncement, has been studying the subject in his laboratory at San Francisco's Langley Porter Institute, where he has found that most people have the wrong impression about how to beat stress. He believes that the common prescription to "take a vacation" or to "ease up at work" have only limited usefulness. When you come back from vacation or slack off at work, he says, you face the same problems with closer deadlines, and as a result, you can become even more tense.

For some people, changing jobs is the right way to avoid stress. For others, though, the answer may lie in streamlining their work, in learning how to pare down social obligations, and in not trying to cram too much into too little time. The feeling of constant pressure at work and at home, and of overwhelming, bone-tired fatigue are among the most common forerunners of heart attack. The only way off this potentially deadly treadmill is to learn how to relax.

Some people find that they can relieve tension by looking out the window and mentally shifting gears or by taking a walk, practicing yoga or stopping to chat with a co-worker.

A quiet environment and a repetitive stimulus such as a single word or phrase repeated over and over in one's mind is the key to the "relaxation response" devised by the Harvard University cardiologist Herbert Benson, M.D., and described in his book by the same title.

In the final analysis, though, if you fit into the Type A category you should ask yourself, as Drs. Friedman and Rosenman advise, "What, apart from the eternal clutter of my everyday living, should be the essence of my life?" The two cardiologists recommend eliminating extraneous duties and allowing for breathing space to enjoy friends, family, "the smell of flowers," and the arts. But most of their suggestions are in the realm of philosophy rather than efficiency—to make a better choice between what is worth doing and what is not.

The value of such an approach has been confirmed by the psychologists Suzanne Kobasa and Salvatore Maddi at the University of Chicago. They have found striking differences between the attitudes of executives who are resistant to stress-related illness and those who are most vulnerable. Men in the resistant group have an uncanny ability to cope with stress by pursuing attainable goals and setting realistic priorities. They consider change a challenge rather than a threat. By contrast, the executives who suffer stress-related illnesses are inclined to stick to their pursuits with a single-mindedness that leaves no room for anybody or anything else. They fear change and feel overwhelmed and powerless to cope with life's major problems.

In the words of the acknowledged father of the stress concept, "There is no ready-made formula which will suit everybody," but "even a gramophone needle which gets into a groove and endlessly reiterates the same sound can snap out of it if you just give it a jerk." Hans Selye wrote those words in 1956, but his analogy is just as true, if not more so, today. A mental tug, in the form of a conscious reminder to relax, is not only good advice but good medicine.

8

HIGH BLOOD PRESSURE

According to the National Heart, Lung and Blood Institute's estimates, 35 million American adults—roughly one in four—have definite hypertension (high blood pressure), requiring drug therapy. And an additional 25 million people have borderline hypertension, requiring regular surveillance and precautionary measures, though not necessarily medication. Estimates from other sources are not quite as staggeringly high, but even so, millions of people who are victims of this disease are unaware that they have it.

Hypertension, the so-called silent disease, is thought to underlie many of the problems that plague the heart.

High blood pressure seems to wreak its worst damage on the delicate inner lining of the coronary arteries, particularly at junctures where they branch into smaller channels. The continuous turbulence of the blood, rushing by under higher-than-normal pressure, promotes the build-up of fibrous, cholesterol-laden plaques if serum cholesterol is elevated, which eventually can produce coronary heart disease.

As health-threatening as this is, the damage is not confined to the coronary arteries alone. The high pressure affects the circulation throughout the body. It can cause any pre-existing weakness in the thin-walled arteries that feed the brain to rupture, causing a paralyzing stroke or worse. In time, if the pressure is not reduced, it can damage the eyes and the kidneys, and weaken the pumping ability of the heart itself.

Blood pressure is a measurement of the force of the blood against the walls of the arteries. Although this force is generated by the heart as it pumps, the actual measurement—the familiar numerical figures of a blood-pressure test—is a reflection of the condition of the arteries through which the blood flows. If the small arteries are under tension and constricted by the muscular bands that wrap around their walls, the blood pressure is high. If the arteries are relaxed, the blood pressure is normal.

The walls of the arteries are elastic, and they expand and contract in rhythm with the heartbeat. With each beat, the pressure rises to its peak and then falls for a fraction of a second as the heart rests between contractions. That's why there are two numbers in a blood-pressure reading. The upper figure (normally between 110 and 140) is a measure of the peak, or systolic, pressure when the heart is contracting, while the lower figure (normally between 60 and 90) is the diastolic pressure when the heart is resting.

Clusters of pressure-sensitive cells in the aorta and carotid arteries automatically monitor the blood pressure, raising it in response to nervous tension or physical exertion, and lowering it when the mood or activity subsides.

When adjustments are necessary, as they frequently are during the day when the body is subjected to emotional stress or when it goes from inactivity to activity, these cells trigger the release of chemical signals that cause millions of still smaller arteries to dilate if the pressure decreases or to constrict if the pressure increases. When the signal says "clamp down," as it does if you are startled, the heart has to pump harder to force the blood through the network of constricted arteries, and this increases the pressure in the circulatory system.

Our blood pressure rises temporarily when we are excited or when our bodies are working very hard. In the latter instance, arteries in the intestine constrict while those that feed the muscles in the limbs dilate and bring additional blood, along with the oxygen and nutrients it carries, to where it is needed most.

Statistical evidence compiled during research over the last two decades shows that high blood pressure tends to cause hardening of the arteries rather than the other way around (though the mechanism for this remains unclear). It was in these studies that the range for normal blood pressure was found to be 110/60 to 140/90. Any consistent at-rest reading above the high figure places the heart and blood vessels in jeopardy. Physicians have found substantial evidence implicating each increment above the normal blood pressure with increased risks for heart failure, strokes and heart attacks (from years of pumping against increased arterial resistance).

Blood pressure

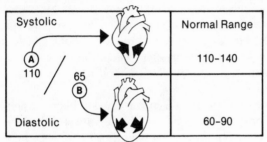

Systolic		Normal Range
(A) 110		110–140
65 (B)		
Diastolic		60–90

Source: *Your Blood Pressure*, © American Medical Association

This potentially lethal association between blood pressure and heart disease may take as long as twenty years to develop, and unlike sudden bacterial infections, hypertension produces no signs or symptoms other than an elevation in blood pressure for the first thirteen or so years of its course. Then it may signal its presence with early-morning headaches or some other, seemingly unrelated symptom.

The only way to tell if you have hypertension is to have your blood pressure checked several times. A single elevated reading does not necessarily mean you have hypertension. Wide fluctuations in blood pressure are, in fact, normal, and if you are anything but calm when you are having the blood-pressure cuff wrapped around your arm and pumped up, your blood pressure will reflect your internal anxiety.

For a true reading, you have to be relaxed. Sometimes, according to Ray W. Gifford, M.D., a leading authority on hypertension at the Cleveland Clinic, this means a second, third or fourth reading on subsequent days. Contrary to popular notions, tense or nervous people are no more hypertensive than others. Nonetheless, some physicians feel that an environment perceived by the individual to be stressful can aggravate a tendency toward hypertension.

Studies of stressful versus less stressful occupations seem to bear this out. Researchers in one often quoted study found that high-pressured air-traffic controllers had four times as much hypertension as did a similar group working in less stressful aviation positions. But the tendency to draw a conclusion from this has to be tempered, as other research has shown, by the possibility that people with a predisposition toward hypertension tend to gravitate to pressure-cooker jobs which require split-second decisions. Thus, the proverbial question about what comes first —the chicken or the egg—persists, and in the case of hypertension, the answer will in all likelihood turn out to be a little of each.

If emotional stress is a factor in causing hypertension, it is not alone. Common everyday salt, birth-control pills, heredity and that old bugaboo, those extra pounds, all have been implicated in the chain of events that produce high blood pressure in the vast majority of people. (An excessive secretion of certain hormones produced by cells in and on top of the kidney can be the source of the trouble, but this rarely occurs.)

Fortunately, if hypertension is detected early enough, it can in almost all instances be controlled before any irreversible damage is done. Since hypertension can develop at any time, it pays to get your blood pressure checked at least once a year. That's the first step. But there are some related conditions you might want to think about:

Is too much salt bad for everyone?

Most of us consume twenty to thirty times more salt a day than the body requires and we simply excrete the excess with no problem at all. But a sizable percentage of people—perhaps 20 to 25 percent—have an inherited inability to handle the excess, and they can develop blood-pressure problems.

The extra salt draws additional fluid into the circulation, which increases the total volume of the blood and also affects the smooth muscle cells of arteries. This, in turn, increases the blood pressure.

A low-salt diet can help reverse the sequence, decreasing the volume and lowering the pressure.

Is excess weight associated with hypertension?

Yes, the extra pounds that come from overeating can dangerously raise the blood pressure. Investigators for the Framingham Study found that a 15 percent gain in weight was accompanied by an 18 percent increase in the systolic pressure. Still other studies have shown that people in their twenties and thirties who are significantly overweight are twice as likely to have hypertension as are people of normal weight.

If you are overweight, you *may* be able to reduce your high blood pressure to normal simply by reducing your weight. In an experiment in Israel, Tel Aviv University Medical School investigators persuaded a group of overweight, hypertensive patients to follow a strict diet that produced an average weight loss of 21 pounds per person over two months. In the same period, blood pressure dropped back into the normal range in 75 percent of the people.

Can emotional stress cause hypertension?

The answer is hazy. While many psychologists think stress is the whole key to hypertension, Cleveland Clinic's Dr. Gifford does not agree. "I think stress plays a role, but how much of a role nobody knows."

As in so many important areas of life, common sense must be our principal guide regarding stress. We know that recreation, relaxation and exercise soothe our spirits, and that sufficient rest and sleep are desirable. We also know that certain situations elevate blood pressure. It may not be possible to prevent hypertension by developing a calmer approach to life or by changing to a less stressful job, but to the extent that such modifications are feasible, they might help.

Do women face any special risks?

Women are as vulnerable to hypertension as men, and in certain circumstances, even more so. Many studies have shown that birth-control pills raise blood pressure *slightly* in almost all women who take them. But some women "on the pill"—perhaps only one in

100—are especially susceptible to developing significant hypertension, which persists even after the pill is stopped, particularly if they have a family history of high blood pressure or if they are overweight.

As a rule, women who have had hypertension should refrain from taking the pill, and women who are susceptible to hypertension—for instance, overweight women—should strongly consider another means of contraception or be given blood-pressure-controlling medicine. All women who consider taking oral contraceptives should have their blood pressure taken when they start using the pill, and every six months thereafter, as the pill's hypertensive effect may be delayed.

During pregnancy, hypertension can develop very rapidly, which is why physicians measure the blood pressure frequently. Also, pre-existing hypertension may become more severe during pregnancy. So it is especially critical to get regular checkups and follow your doctor's advice during this period.

Women whose blood pressure has been normal all their lives need to pay special attention to it after menopause and should have it checked at least once a year. After her childbearing years are over, a woman's risk of hypertension becomes greater than a man's. A postmenopausal woman on estrogen therapy, which is similar in its effects to oral contraceptives, should have her blood pressure checked at least every six months.

What happens if a doctor discovers high blood pressure?

Don't be alarmed—it can often be treated effectively with simple measures that work. Stick to one reliable, interested physician or one good clinic, and follow through with the treatment plan, which may include changes in lifestyle, diet and physical activity.

Most hypertension therapy begins with a reduction in salt intake and with weight control. Sometimes this is enough. In other instances a diuretic medication may be prescribed to stimulate the excretion of excess salt. For at least one third of the people with mild hypertension, this is the only treatment needed to reduce the blood pressure to normal. Frequently the diuretic makes it unnecessary to undertake a rigid low-salt diet—2 grams or less of salt a day—which some people find bland and difficult to follow. Almost all diuretics remove potassium from the body, so potassium-rich foods such as orange juice, raisins, bananas and dried fruits, or even potassium tablets, may be recommended.

Many physicians treat hypertension in a stepped-care approach. This means starting with a small dose of one drug, usually a diuretic, increasing it if necessary, and then adding other, more powerful drugs as needed.

If weight seems to be the major problem, the physician might begin antihypertensive medication promptly, while at the same time recommending weight loss, a low-salt diet and exercise. If the patient loses weight, the drug dosage may be tapered off or even eliminated. Such treatment spares the heart and arteries from the stress of high blood pressure during the often lengthy period that might be required to lose weight. On the other hand, if the hypertension is not severe, the doctor might suggest a low-calorie diet before he decides whether or not to prescribe drugs. This leeway in treatment permits individualized regimens, and your doctor will choose from among the various approaches the one that will work best for you.

Are there any pitfalls associated with the treatment?

Not with the treatment, but the biggest danger is that you will become bored or complacent and stop taking your medicine once your blood pressure has dropped to normal. A few years ago it was estimated that only one in seven hypertensive Americans was following an adequate regimen program. One solution to this has been the growing tendency of physicians to train their patients or their patient's family members to take their blood pressure at home. If you see for yourself how your blood pressure remains low while you are taking the medication, you may have more incentive to stay with it.

Remember: Hypertension is usually a lifelong condition, and the treatment must continue even after it brings the blood pressure down to normal. The disease itself may be silent, but the message is loud and clear. A "mild" case of hypertension can double your chances of heart attack, and a "moderate" case can triple them. Unless the trouble is caught and treated, it will steadily erode the heart's reserves and corrode vital arteries. So roll up your sleeve, relax, and have your blood pressure taken. It is painless, and it could save your life.

9

SMOKING

Elizabeth I, the daughter of Henry VIII and Anne Boleyn, had been Queen of England for twenty-eight years when one of her ships, fresh from a voyage to the New World, dropped anchor with a new and unique cargo of expensive dry leaves gathered from colonies in Virginia. The year was 1586, and the shipment was the first of many to come of a plant that would later be scientifically classified as *Nicotiana tabacum.* Tobacco had come to Europe.

The use of the chopped and finely ground leaves in pipes and as snuff flourished during Elizabeth's reign, and by the year of her death, in 1603, when James I ascended the throne, tobacco had become a fixture at court among the fashionable and wealthy. It is not recorded which ministers had James's ear or whether they turned him against tobacco, but in 1604 he decried its use and condemned it as "that outlandish weed."

He was the first of many to see a lurking danger through the veil of smoke. Today practically everyone has heard that smoking is unhealthy. This is the message that the Surgeon General and other physicians have been trying to get across for years, but they are having as difficult a time penetrating the public mind as James I did. Millions of people blithely ignore the warning and continue to smoke.

Mike B., a sales manager for most of his life, was like many people in this respect. He was accustomed to reading reports that cigarettes shorten one's life, but he never took the message personally. He always thought that the statistics would catch up with someone else.

When he was forty-five years old Mike suffered a heart attack, which his doctor attributed at least in part to his having smoked two to three packs of cigarettes a day since he was sixteen. When Mike was told that there was a connection between his smoking habits and his damaged heart, he was astonished. Many smokers have a similar reaction. They do not realize that smoking cigarettes is *more likely* to cause heart disease than it is to cause lung cancer.

It is estimated that cigarette smoking is responsible for more than 300,000 deaths each year. Of these, 19 percent are due to lung cancer, but 37 percent—i.e., nearly twice as many—result from coronary heart disease. The doctor who attended Mike told him this and advised him in no uncertain terms to give up the habit. Despite the warning, though, Mike clung to the smoker's most dangerous myth. As he expressed it two years later, shortly before his death from a second heart attack: "I figured, what the hell, I've smoked all these years and the damage is done. I might as well light up and enjoy the rest of my life. It's too late to quit."

Although a great many heart-attack victims actually are frightened into quitting cigarettes for good, others are so blinded by an apparent "death wish" that, like Mike, they fail to absorb the single most important point about stopping the habit—that *it is almost never too late to quit.* Within days after the last lungful of cigarette smoke, the body begins to repair itself. Harmful chemicals from cigarettes no longer circulate through the bloodstream, the lungs begin to clear, and the smoke-impaired senses of taste and smell begin to revive.

Despite the frustration caused by breaking an addiction to nicotine, many people who have stopped smoking notice almost immediately that they have more energy, sleep better and in general feel better. Within a year, according to a National Cancer Institute study of more than a million people, an ex-smoker's risk of heart attack plummets. The risk of lung cancer starts dropping after two years. And after ten smoke-free years, a person who formerly consumed a pack or less a day has the same mortality risk as someone who has never smoked.

Cigarettes do their damage through the products of combustion that are drawn into the lungs. Tar and nicotine are only the best-known of the numerous hazardous components of cigarettes that diffuse throughout a smoker's body. Nearly 90 percent of cigarette smoke consists of a dozen harmful gases, including hydrogen cyanide, a deadly poison that damages the lining of the lungs, and nitrogen oxide, a compound that robs the lungs of their elasticity and contributes to emphysema. But the gas most closely associated with heart disease is carbon monoxide, the same colorless, odorless compound that makes automobile exhaust fumes deadly.

Carbon monoxide in the lungs competes with oxygen for space inside the red blood cells, which act as a transport system to carry the gases to every cell in the body. It is similar to a crowd of people pushing and shoving to get into a subway car. But because of specific chemical forces, carbon monoxide always wins out. Whenever carbon monoxide is present in the lungs, it will latch on to the molecular "hooks" that are normally reserved for oxygen in the red blood cells. This decreases the amount of oxygen that can be carried by red blood cells and also slows down the release of the remaining oxygen to the tissues. Respiratory physiologists now know that this is one reason why even a young smoker may feel winded after climbing a flight or two of stairs.

Depending upon the number and brand of cigarettes smoked, a person may displace 10 to 15 percent of the oxygen in his bloodstream with carbon monoxide. The body partially compensates by manufacturing more red blood cells. But the nicotine in cigarette smoke diminishes the effectiveness of this internal balance by making the heart work harder and, therefore, use up even more oxygen than it ordinarily does.

Nicotine is one of a number of naturally occurring, addictive plant compounds, including opium and cocaine, that produce changes inside the human body. When a cigarette is lit, some of the nicotine is burned, some is trapped by the filter (if it is a filtered brand), but appreciable quantities get into the system through the lung's air sacs and produce measurable changes almost immediately. Under the prodding of nicotine, the adrenal glands (which sit atop the kidneys) and certain heart tissues release powerful stimulants known as catecholamines, principally composed of adrenalin, which start the smoker's heart pounding an extra fifteen to twenty-five beats per minute. The catecholamines also constrict small arteries throughout the body, elevating blood pressure by as much as twenty points.

This combination of a faster heart rate and higher blood pressure causes the heart muscle to work harder and consume more oxygen. The trouble is that carbon monoxide—from the same lungful of smoke that brought in nicotine—reduces the oxygen supply. A smoker's body can adjust by shifting blood toward the heart and away from less vital organs and tissues. In a heart already damaged by coronary artery disease, however, this may not be enough. Caught in the two-fisted grip of nicotine stimulation and a temporary shortage of oxygen, the heart may signal its distress with the chest discomfort of angina pectoris.

If cigarette smoking could affect the heart's rate and oxygen supply, then in all probability it is associated with heart attacks. This is precisely what researchers have determined. The association is so close, in fact, that smoking turns out to be the *number-one* risk factor for heart attacks, ranking above high serum cholesterol and hypertension. In large-scale studies, these researchers found that smokers with normal cholesterol levels and normal blood pressure and none of the other risk factors for heart disease are 70 percent more likely to die of a heart attack than similarly healthy nonsmokers.

Carbon monoxide, they found, not only reduces the oxygen-carrying capacity of the blood but also hurts circulation by making the walls of arteries more permeable—opening minute pores in the arterial walls, which produces edema (an abnormal accumulation of fluid) in the walls. This, in turn, can promote the deposition of cholesterol in the arterial walls. Autopsies of heavy smokers in this country reveal that their arteries are generally harder and thicker due to atherosclerosis than those of nonsmokers.

Many researchers now believe that it is the combination of carbon monoxide and elevated cholesterol levels that makes cigarette smoking such an important risk factor for coronary disease in this country. According to University of Chicago's Dr. Wissler, smoking does not seem to promote coronary heart disease until the blood cholesterol level goes above 150. When it goes above 200—a level that is not unusual in the average American adult—statistical evidence shows a strong link between smoking and the disease process that clogs coronary arteries.

On top of this effect, smoking is also known to increase the clotting ability of blood, in part by acting on platelets—the minute cell fragments in the blood which normally clump together to patch over a wounded area. But in arteries narrowed by fatty deposits, clotting of the platelets may form a plug that blocks the artery. If it is a coronary artery that is blocked, the result is a heart attack.

The clotting factor in cigarette smoke, according to one theory, is a tobacco substance known as rutin, which causes an allergic reaction that promotes clotting in certain smokers. Tests at New York–Cornell Medical College found 12 of 31 volunteers to be sensitive to rutin. The Cornell pathologist Carl G. Becker, M.D., speculates that sensitivity of the heart muscle to certain elements in cigarette smoke, including rutin, may disrupt the heart's normally smooth rhythm. This, in turn, may decrease the heart's ability to move blood through its chambers and impair the blood flow through the coronary arteries. If Dr. Becker's theory is correct, it would help to account for the high susceptibility of smokers to sudden death from heart attack.

Since the first Surgeon General's Report on Smoking and Health, in 1964, the percentage of men who smoke has dropped from 52 percent to 39 percent, and this has been paralleled by a decline in the death rate from smoking-related diseases such as chronic bronchitis and emphysema. But the percentage of teenage girls who smoke has increased, and the percentage of women who smoke has stayed almost the same. It is an ominous sign of the times that the death rate from lung diseases among women has increased, led by the lung-cancer rates, which have doubled. Health experts fear that this is only the tip of an ugly iceberg, reflecting an upsurge in smoking by women who started the habit in the 1950s and 1960s, decades later than men.

Women are now smoking at an earlier age than before, thus increasing the total number of cigarettes consumed in a lifetime. In 1968, only half as many girls as boys aged twelve to eighteen smoked at least once a week, 9 percent versus 17 percent. But by 1974 the smoking rates were virtually the same, 15.3 percent for girls and 15.8 percent for boys. If the same pattern holds true for

women as it has for men—and there is no reason to suspect that
it will not—the cumulative damage to women's hearts from years
of smoking will also begin taking its toll before many more years
have passed.

For women who take birth-control pills, the situation is especially alarming. Smoking and the pill are a dangerous combination
that significantly increases a woman's risk of suffering a heart
attack. A study by Anrudh K. Jain of the Population Council done
in the late 1970s revealed that the mortality rate from heart attack
is about six times as high among women who smoke and use the
pill as among nonsmokers who use the pill.

The vulnerability of a woman's body to damage from smoking
extends, if she is pregnant, to her unborn baby as well. Smoking
cuts down the flow of oxygen and nutrients to the womb, thus
hampering the baby's growth. In a study in Israel, babies born to
mothers who smoked throughout pregnancy were found to weigh
an average of seven ounces less than those born to nonsmoking
mothers. According to the American Cancer Society, smoking
mothers have twice the number of miscarriages and stillbirths as
have nonsmoking mothers. Also, their babies are more likely to
become ill or die than in cases where the mothers do not smoke.

One of the most revealing facts about cigarettes is the number
of smokers who would like to give them up. If all the people who
say they would like to quit actually did so, the single most preventable cause of heart disease—in the words of the American Heart
Association—would become a minor threat to public health. Nine
out of ten smokers interviewed in a Gallup poll taken in the
mid-1970s had at some time tried to stop smoking or indicated they
would do so if they could find an easy method.

Happily, more than 30 million Americans have found a way.
And more than 95 percent of them, it is estimated, have quit
smoking on their own—without resorting to psychiatrists, medication or self-help groups. According to Donald R. Shopland,
technical information officer of the United States Public Health
Service Office on Smoking and Health, the most successful
method has proved to be the simplest: "cold turkey"—stopping
completely rather than tapering off. Not surprisingly, light smokers and people worried about their health have been the most
successful in stopping.

Still, that leaves some 50 million Americans who are locked into the cigarette habit. For them, perhaps the chief obstacle to a personal decision to stop smoking is the belief that quitting involves a sacrifice, a net loss. Any smoker who believes that the satisfactions of smoking outweigh the benefits of quitting ought to add up the unpleasant things connected with the habit. The list is a long one, and it includes throat irritation, morning cough, a loss of taste and smell, and the prospect of crippling bronchitis or emphysema in later life—not to mention the threat of lung cancer and heart disease.

If that is not enough, consider these answers to some of the most common questions—and misconceptions—about smoking:

Are today's filter cigarettes a lot safer than the ones people used to smoke?

Filters are cutting the risk of lung cancer by reducing tar. But even so, the filter smoker is still four times as likely to develop this disease as is the nonsmoker. And two studies, one conducted in England and one in the United States, suggest that filter cigarettes may actually *increase* the danger of heart disease by allowing carbon monoxide to build up in the blood. The reason is that filter cigarettes are harder to draw on, so less oxygen is pulled into the lungs with each breath than with an easier-drawing cigarette. The less oxygen brought to the lungs in a breath, the more carbon monoxide remains in the blood. However, if the filter cigarette is perforated around the tip, as a few brands are, that difference is eliminated.

What about low-tar, low-nicotine cigarettes?

An American Cancer Society study of a million people between 1960 and 1972 showed substantially lower death rates for those who smoked low-tar, low-nicotine cigarettes as compared with those who smoked stronger brands. But the death rate among the "safer" smokers is still 30 to 75 percent higher than among nonsmokers.

Does the number of cigarettes smoked have anything to do with heart disease?

Yes, the fewer cigarettes smoked, the lower the risk of heart

This Pump Beats 100,000 Times a Day

Your heart, which is about the size of your fist, pumps 2,000 gallons of blood a day through your circulatory system. Used blood (blue) returns from body via veins (1) to the right atrium (2). When the atrium has filled, it contracts, squishing blood through valve (3) into right ventricle (4). Valve closes as ventricle pumps blood through pulmonary artery (5) to lungs (6), where it is oxygenated. Oxygenated blood (red) reverts along pulmonary veins (7) to left atrium (8). Atrium pushes blood through mitral valve (9) to thick-walled left ventricle (10). This powerful, muscular ventricle then pumps blood through aorta (11) to body and to coronary arteries. (The latter feed the heart itself.) Both atria (2,8) contract in unison, alternating rhythmically with ventricles (4,10) about 70 times per minute.

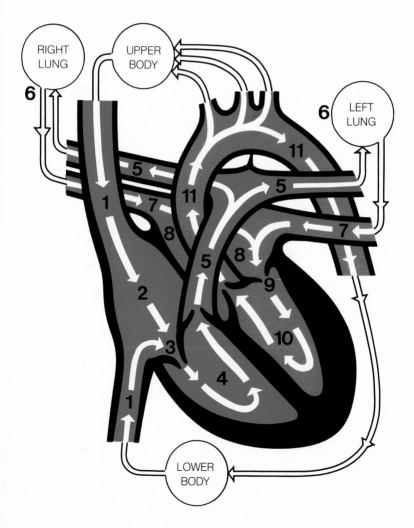

A 60,000-Mile Network of Blood Vessels

Like a tree with many branches, the blood vessels diverge from the heart (generalized area outlined in black) to smaller pipelines and tubes. The arteries (red) carry oxygen-rich blood from the heart to all the organs of the body. The veins subsequently return the oxygen-depleted blood to the heart where the fluid is replenished with oxygen, in a continuing cycle of nourishment. In all, it is estimated that there are 60,000 miles of arteries, arterioles, capillaries, venules and veins comprising your body's vascular system.

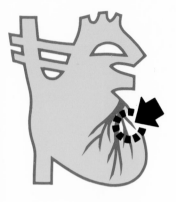

Warning: Heart Attack Ahead

Though a heart attack strikes in seconds, the groundwork for it often takes years. The gradual deterioration of coronary vessels leads to reduced blood supply (see cross-sectional diagrams below) and, finally, to the destruction of myocardial tissue. Heart attacks can strike any part of the heart, but the most frequent target is the front left area served by the left anterior coronary artery (see illustration at left).

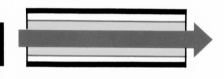

Blood (red) flows through healthy open coronary artery (yellow).

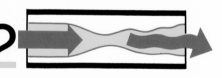

Fatty deposits roughen and narrow the interior surface of the artery, causing degeneration and narrowing of the artery, and reduced blood flow.

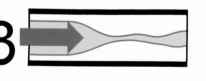

Vessels are now so narrow and rigid that barely a trickle of blood can pass through.

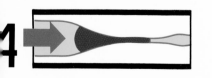

Here we see the final blockage of the artery, which is caused by a blood clot that has formed in the narrowed vessel.

The Body Fights to Save Itself

When the coronary arteries (yellow) are open and healthy, blood (red) flows through them freely like traffic moving along the lanes of a freeway.

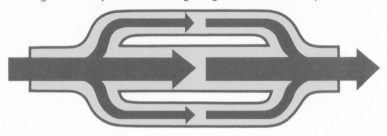

Over the years, however, fat and other debris may harden and block the main vessel (gray area). The stage is now set for a heart attack. Fighting to save itself, the body may seek a way to bypass the blockage.

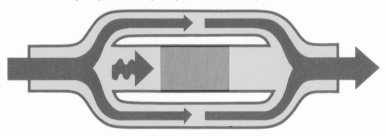

In this example, the side lanes enlarge to provide collateral circulation. Rapid development of the collateral vessels decreases the load on the clogged main vessel, thereby endeavoring to head off the heart attack. When physicians feel that this natural process may not be sufficient to prevent a heart attack, bypass surgery is sometimes performed.

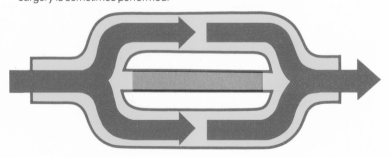

disease for the average American. The trick comes in maintaining a low level of smoking.

Short of going "cold turkey," what method of quitting cigarettes is best?

One of the most successful methods is the eight-step technique suggested by the American Cancer Society. Many of the smoking withdrawal clinics rely on the same or similar steps:

1. List your reasons for and against smoking.
2. Change to a low-tar, low-nicotine cigarette (if you do not already smoke them) and select a Q (quit) Day, which is an arbitrary date, let's say three weeks or a month away.
3. Chart your smoking habits for at least two weeks. Write down how many cigarettes you smoke a day and when you smoke them. Go over this list and rank which cigarette you think is the most important or desirable to you, such as the one with morning coffee; the next most important one; and so on down to the least important.
4. Eliminate one of the cigarettes you routinely smoke. It may be the most important one, or the one in the middle of your list, or the least important one.
5. Secure a supply of "oral substitutes": mints, gum, an inhaler, ginger root, or even mouthwash, and use it instead of reaching for a cigarette.
6. Repeat each night, at least ten times, one of your reasons for not smoking.
7. Quit on Q Day. Try different substitutes as the urge to smoke recurs. Enlist your spouse or a friend in a series of busy events, such as going to the movies or theater, playing tennis, taking several long walks.
8. Keep reminding yourself, again and again, of the shocking risks of cigarette smoking.

Is one "stop-smoking clinic" program better than another?

The question is almost impossible to answer as so much depends upon the original motivation of those who participate in a given method. "If people plunk down two hundred and fifty dollars to stop smoking," explains one leader of a nonprofit program, "that in itself is a powerful incentive to stop. But whether the expensive programs are any better, per se, than a course for ten dollars, I don't know."

If you need help to find a stop-smoking clinic, ask your family physician or contact your local chapter of the American Cancer Society, the American Heart Association, or the American Lung Association.

How successful are self-help groups and counseling?

Smoking-withdrawal clinics, which offer tips on how to quit and reinforce the smoker's desire to stop, and individual counseling, which basically takes the same route, produce abstinence rates of 20 to 35 percent one year after treatment. That success rate is not as dismal as it sounds. Many of the people who seek help from therapists and clinics are difficult cases who have tried and failed to quit on their own. Furthermore, the person who fails with one method can always try another and perhaps succeed on a second or third try.

What is "aversion therapy"?

This is a series of conditioning routines designed to produce an automatic, psychological reaction against smoking by instantly associating it with unpleasant things. The key techniques used in this type of therapy include rapid smoking, in which the subject inhales every six seconds or so until he can no longer tolerate the smoke; daily sessions in front of a machine that blows smoke directly into the smoker's face; and the administration of mild electric shocks every time the subject lights a cigarette. Because of the possible dangers involved in rapid smoking, these programs should have tight medical controls and electroencephalogram (EEG) monitoring, especially for anyone with a history of cardiovascular disease, high blood pressure, diabetes or respiratory disease.

Can the smoking habit be stopped by hypnosis?

There is disagreement among the experts on this subject. Some believe that hypnosis works for one smoker in five, but others claim that it only succeeds with people who are so determined that they would be able to quit on their own. In any event, it is not a sure-fire method.

Are there any drugs that can take away the urge for a cigarette?

Over-the-counter preparations containing the drug lobeline have been marketed as aids to smokers who want to quit, but these preparations are actually no more effective than placebos or sugar pills in reducing the desire to smoke. If you are considering using a lobeline-type drug, you may want to consult your family physician for his assessment of its effectiveness and his recommendation. In general, it is advisable to take as few drugs as possible. If you do take them, read the labels and instructions carefully.

Is cigarette smoke in the air harmful to people who don't smoke?

Yes, it can be. Children of smokers have been shown to have more respiratory illnesses than children of nonsmokers. In a smoke-filled room, it is possible for a nonsmoker to inhale the equivalent of one cigarette per hour.

It is possible to ignore all the evidence on the harmful side of smoking. Millions of people do it every day when they light up. But sooner or later, the lung and heart diseases that come from cigarettes will not ignore the smoker.

10

ESPECIALLY FOR DIABETICS

In January 1968, in an operating room at the Groote Schuur Hospital in Capetown, South Africa, a surgeon made history by successfully transplanting a human heart. Reports of the dramatic feat made headlines in newspapers around the world, and the doctor and his patient came for a time under the close scrutiny of the public eye. Every move either of them made was dutifully documented, no matter how seemingly insignificant. Yet one fact was nearly overlooked. The patient, Philip Blaiberg, D.D.S., who went on to live 563 days with the transplanted heart, had diabetes mellitus.

This disease probably had little or no effect on the processes within Dr. Blaiberg's body that finally caused the donor "foreign" heart to be rejected. But diabetes undoubtedly was an important factor in the condition crippling Dr. Blaiberg's own heart, making Dr. Christiaan Barnard's heroic surgery necessary in the first place.

Diabetes is more than simply the blood-sugar disorder that it was thought to be for centuries. Although it certainly affects the amount of sugar in the blood, it also may injure the blood vessels themselves, eventually causing leakage in the capillaries in the eyes, in the kidneys and in the heart. Some researchers speculate that the genetic defect that produces diabetes also causes the changes in blood-vessel walls. Others ascribe the capillary damage to increased levels of blood sugar, although just how this injures the vessels is unclear. And still others wonder if the combination of elevated blood sugar and elevated blood cholesterol is at the root of the vascular problem.

No matter which theory eventually proves correct—and they are all being intensively investigated—it is a medical fact that diabetes damages blood vessels and that damaged blood vessels are susceptible to atherosclerosis. If the blood-vessel damage in the eyes is not detected and treated early enough, blurred vision and even blindness can result. When blood vessels in the kidneys are affected, the blood flow within this impaired organ is reduced. The kidneys are very sensitive to blood flow; they need a steady, normal supply of blood to function properly. When the flow is reduced, they try to rectify the situation by increasing the blood pressure through a system of enzymes and hormones that constrict other blood vessels in the body. A type of kidney cells, called juxtaglomerular cells, produce the enzyme renin in increased quantities when the blood flow to the kidneys is reduced. This enzyme activates a substance called angiotensin, produced by the liver. Angiotensin, in turn, causes constriction in the walls of arteries, thereby increasing the blood pressure.

In the case of diabetes, the blood flow to the kidneys may be permanently reduced due to the damage the disease causes to blood vessels in the organ. This can lead to hypertension, among other disorders. But the most life-threatening of the vascular disorders that plague diabetics is accelerated atherosclerosis, particularly in the coronary arteries, as well as in the arteries that supply the brain.

The process of atherosclerosis may take decades in the case of a nondiabetic before it affects the heart or the brain. But in a person whose blood vessels have been damaged by diabetes, it has been found to occur much more quickly; and that is why diabetics face a greater risk than nondiabetics of heart attacks and strokes. Diabetes alone—without any other heart-attack risk factors—doubles a man's susceptibility to cardiovascular disease, and triples a woman's susceptibility. When other risk factors are present, a diabetic's chances of suffering a heart attack keep multiplying.

According to statistical evidence from the Framingham Study, if a forty-year-old man with diabetes also has high serum cholesterol, he raises his risk of heart disease eight times above that of a diabetic with normal cholesterol. And if he smokes cigarettes as well, his risk will be more than eleven times as high. It was a combination of risk factors on top of diabetes that impaired the function of Philip Blaiberg's heart to the point that it could no longer keep him alive, even though it continued to beat feebly the morning of the historic operation.

Fortunately, evidence suggests that diabetics can ward off heart damage by using methods that physicians recommend to control diabetes itself. If the disorder is kept in check by a combination of drugs (if they are necessary), proper diet and exercise, a diabetic's prospect of getting coronary heart disease is not significantly worse than the nondiabetic's.

Some four million Americans are afflicted with diabetes, although only half that number are aware that they have it. That's because the disorder can come on slowly and insidiously in some people, producing few if any symptoms at first. Or it can strike swiftly and dramatically, necessitating prompt medical attention. In either instance, the blood sugar called glucose begins to accumulate in the circulatory system rather than enter cells where it is used to fuel the metabolic machinery that keeps tissues and organs functioning normally.

The major regulator of the glucose supply is insulin, a hormone produced by specialized cells within the pancreas. In a healthy nondiabetic, insulin is automatically released to keep the proper amount of glucose in the blood. But either diabetics do not produce sufficient insulin or, if they actually do produce some, their cells cannot utilize it to absorb glucose from the blood.

Excess glucose causes changes in almost every organ of the body. And these changes, in turn, produce the main symptoms of diabetes: increased thirst from dehydration, frequent urination, and weight loss in spite of an increased appetite. Occasionally these symptoms are ignored when people simply pass them off as signs of growing older or as the lingering effects of a bad cold. Doctors frequently discover diabetes in patients who complain of blurred vision, or a loss of sensation in the skin, or a bothersome sore on the leg or foot. Simple tests for sugar in the urine and blood are all that is needed to make an unequivocal diagnosis.

Physicians have found one additional wrinkle in the diagnosis of diabetes, and this is usually related to a person's age. If the disorder strikes in childhood or during the young adult years it is called juvenile diabetes. Although only 10 percent of diabetics have this form of the disorder, it is more serious because little or no insulin is produced and therefore daily injections of the hormone are necessary. Since diabetes tends to run in families, children should be tested regularly if one of their parents or grandparents or any other close relative has this disorder.

Two genes among the thousands that determine our heredity are thought to carry the weakness for the disorder. But these genes by themselves may not be the whole cause of the problem. Researchers believe that some kind of "trigger" is necessary to start the insulin-deficiency process. Outbreaks of juvenile diabetes have followed epidemics of childhood diseases, particularly mumps (for which there is now a vaccine), and there is speculation that a virus may instigate the disorder, either by destroying the insulin-producing cells in the pancreas or by stimulating the diabetes-prone genes.

With present methods of treatment, juvenile diabetics can lead relatively normal lives, although in the past their life expectancy was about 30 percent shorter than that of the nondiabetic. This makes juvenile diabetes a harsher foe than the variety of the disorder that strikes older people, known as adult-onset diabetes. As the name implies, this form of diabetes usually strikes in middle age, most often when the victim is in his fifties or sixties.

About 90 percent of all diabetics suffer from the adult-onset form, and most of them usually do not require insulin injections because they produce enough of the hormone. Their trouble lies in an inability to use the insulin properly. Although there is no cure for diabetes, the sugar level of their blood can be kept within normal limits by diet, exercise and weight reduction, and these three remedies hold the key to decreasing their risk of heart disease.

This was the lesson Jim Bissel learned when he was forty-eight years old and appeared at his doctor's office for his annual physical. During a routine test the doctor discovered sugar in Jim's urine and asked him to return the next day for a glucose tolerance test. Following an overnight fast and an initial blood test, Jim swallowed a large glass of a drink heavily sweetened with glucose. The objective: to find out how his body handled a massive dose of sugar.

Several times during the next three hours a medical assistant took a sample of Jim's blood and analyzed it for sugar. The level was clearly elevated, indicating that his body was not handling sugar in the normal way. If he had been normal, his body would have stored the fuel for later use by converting it into glycogen in the liver, and the sugar level in his blood would have stayed within a certain range during the testing period, despite the heavy load of glucose he had swallowed.

Most adult-onset diabetics are overweight, and Jim was no exception. Excess fat, it is theorized, makes cells in many tissues of the body somewhat resistant to insulin, which would otherwise act as a sort of catalyst in helping the cells to absorb glucose from the bloodstream. When excess weight is lost, this insulin resistance may diminish.

Unlike diabetic diets in the past, which sharply limited starches, the modern diets are not nearly as restrictive. Most diabetics can consume about 45 percent of their total calories from bread, potatoes and pasta—a total that is approximately the same as in the nondiabetic diet. The main dietary ingredient for adult-onset diabetics to avoid is refined sugar in all its forms. This means no pies, cakes, soft drinks or candy.

Exercise is also an important part of a weight-control, heart-strengthening program, as mentioned in a previous chapter. But for a diabetic it has an extra benefit. Exercise tends to accelerate the entry of glucose into muscle cells, and by itself it can lower the blood-sugar level. In fact, those diabetics who are dependent on insulin injections usually have to cut their dosage by 10 to 30 percent during a day of vigorous activity. Jim Bissell, following his doctor's advice, jogs every morning, and this activity, combined with his diet, has kept his weight in check and has made it unnecessary for him to continue with the oral diabetes medication that had been prescribed to lower his blood sugar.

In many ways Jim is a typical adult-onset diabetic who has learned to live with his disease and perhaps is even healthier despite it. His cholesterol is down and his hypertension is kept under control with medication. Hence the risk factors that he might have lived with are now virtually eliminated, and the outlook for his future health is sounder than it was when his diabetes was first diagnosed. "The disease," he says, "has affected my life only in a minor way. I am doing the same things—working, socializing, taking trips, sitting at my office desk—as I would be if I didn't have diabetes. I worried about the diagnosis when I first heard it, but ten years later I can honestly say that it hasn't been bad. I simply have had to give up a few old habits and establish a few new ones."

The adjustment is not quite as simple for all diabetics, particularly those with the juvenile-onset form of the disease. They need to follow a far stricter regimen in order to avoid as much as possible the eye, kidney and heart complications. This includes daily insulin injections, daily urinary sugar tests, a regular eating schedule and quick access to a source of sugar in case they feel an attack of low blood sugar coming on. The jolt of insulin from the daily injections can cause a rapid lowering of blood sugar, dropping the level below normal and causing weakness and dizziness, the twin signs of too little glucose in the bloodstream. To counterbalance the drain on their system they have to bring some sugar back into the blood by eating a sugary snack or a piece of candy.

Despite the attention they have to pay to their disease, juvenile-onset diabetics are usually not strapped or hindered in any way from leading normal lives. Few people realize, for instance, that Mary Tyler Moore, the energetic and talented star of many successful television programs, is afflicted with the severe juvenile form of diabetes which she first learned about at the relatively late age of thirty. Her activity—dancing, singing, working very hard as an actress—may have suppressed her blood sugar, masking the symptoms of the disease, which usually appear at an earlier age. Nevertheless, her diabetes surfaced while she was in the hospital after a miscarriage. Pregnancy sometimes brings out a case of "hidden diabetes," which may eventually vanish. But in Mary's case, tests showed that her blood-sugar level did not drop after her miscarriage. In fact, it remained extremely high—750 mg per 100 ml of blood instead of the normal 70 mg to 100 mg per 100 ml, as measured in a blood sample. And the diagnosis of juvenile diabetes was made, even though she was five or so years beyond the upper-limit age at which this form of the disease ordinarily strikes. Consequently, daily insulin injections were prescribed, and she was placed on a strict diet.

If the disease has slowed her down, it certainly is not noticeable.

"I may be kidding myself," she told Caroline Stevens in an interview for *Diabetes Forecast*, "but I really feel I'm probably better off having diabetes than the average person who doesn't have it. I've been told that the life span of someone with diabetes is shorter, but I think I've increased mine with the diet I eat and the exercise I get. So it will probably all even out."

Based on the progress medicine is making in analyzing and treating diabetes, there appears to be solid justification for Mary Tyler Moore's optimism. As this is written, researchers are working to perfect a glucose sensor that will automatically monitor sugar levels when implanted into a diabetic's body. The device first measures glucose levels in the fluid that surrounds the body's internal tissues and then sends a signal to a pocket-sized receiver that displays a numerical figure on a small screen similar to that of a pocket calculator. By checking this figure every now and then, a diabetic with an implanted sensor will be able to adjust his diet or insulin dosage to attain normal, or close-to-normal, blood-sugar levels throughout the day, instead of using the less accurate urine-test–insulin-injection method.

Such glucose sensors are a key element in what researchers call a "bionic pancreas," a still-investigational device that duplicates the two main functions of normal pancreatic insulin-secreting cells—namely, detecting increased glucose levels and dispensing the proper amount of insulin automatically. Besides a glucose sensor, the "bionic pancreas" has a microcomputer for precise calculation of the insulin required to maintain the diabetic's blood sugar within normal range, and a delivery pump to inject the exact dosage.

Other researchers are concentrating on *growing* the insulin-producing pancreatic cells. The rationale behind this line of research is "Why bother to build an artificial pancreas that simulates the activity of the pancreas when the actual thing can be grown in the laboratory?" Not only have insulin-producing cells from animals been grown successfully in the laboratory, but they have been reimplanted into diabetic animals with successful results. The main catch is that the cells, not long after they are implanted, are rejected in the same way many transplanted organs are. To prevent the body's immunity system from recognizing the cells as foreign and rejecting them, the researchers are considering encapsulating the laboratory-grown cells in an artificial membrane that they hope will protect them from immune rejections.

In another line of attack on the disease, a pair of Wisconsin physicians has devised a highly sensitive test that can detect and distinguish between two distinct categories of adult-onset diabetes. Roger W. Turkington, M.D., and Howard K. Weindling, M.D., working with a radioimmunoassay test in Milwaukee's St. Francis Hospital, discovered that half of their 334 adult-onset diabetes patients were producing *normal* quantities of insulin and none of them was suffering from the eye, kidney or heart complications characteristic of the ordinary diabetic. Such people are not diabetics in the true sense of the word, according to Turkington and Weindling. Writing in the *Journal of the American Medical Association*, they have recommended replacement of the time-honored glucose-tolerance test with the inexpensive and widely available radioimmunoassay test. The use of the newer test will enable physicians to better classify—and treat—their diabetic patients. Those who are producing normal or near-normal amounts of insulin could be managed with weight control, diet and exercise, while those who are insulin-deficient could then be promptly started on a permanent series of insulin injections, decreasing their likelihood of future complications.

Methods to combat the disease and refinements in diagnosis are, of course, not synonymous with a cure, but the advances that have already been made, and those that will be coming out of the laboratory in the near future, are making an impact in reducing the potentially damaging complications that threaten a diabetic's heart and longevity.

PART II

11

WHEN SOMETHING GOES WRONG

Writing in *Scientific American* in late 1980, Reuel A. Stallones, M.D., a public health expert at the University of Texas, made a prediction about coronary artery disease and heart attacks that reinforces the main point of the preceding chapters. "The brightest prospects for the future," he wrote, "lie in the effective prevention of the disease." It is never too late to change certain potentially harmful lifestyle habits that have been found to be associated with heart disease by hundreds of medical experts.

No matter how many risk factors you or any member of your family have, you should not be fatalistic about your chances of developing heart disease. In most cases you can measurably improve your chances of avoiding it, as other people have before you. The risk factors discussed in the preceding chapters are the distillation of years of painstaking research, and these conclusions represent hard-won knowledge from scores of scientific studies involving thousands of people. Along with this knowledge have come advances in the diagnosis and treatment of heart disease itself.

Yet coronary disease is, unfortunately, still very much with us. Heart attacks alone account for a third of all deaths in the United States, making heart disease, despite its reduced incidence, still the single greatest cause of death in this country.

When something goes wrong in the heart, what are the symptoms and how can the damage be repaired? These and many related questions have been asked since the early days of cardiology, and even prior to that time. Aside from finding out what causes heart disease and how to prevent it, physicians have developed methods and medications to alleviate suffering, save lives and sometimes restore hearts that are in jeopardy.

Surgeons, using techniques to look inside the living heart, can pinpoint the trouble and go safely into the stilled heart to correct it with artificial parts while a heart-lung machine takes over the pumping work of the heart to keep the brain and the rest of the body supplied with fresh oxygen. This is the most dramatic kind of surgery, unimaginable two or three decades ago, when the interior of the heart was beyond all but a few specially skilled and bold surgeons. Now, with finely crafted laboratory drugs, synthetic vessels, artificial parts and long-lasting pacemakers, the era of heart repair is truly achieving remarkable results.

The diseases that affect the heart may still be devastating—there is no denying that—but the medical and surgical countereffort has made enormous strides, strides in skill, care and compassion that are recounted in the following chapters from the annals of actual cases of people who have been through it.

12

THE HEART ATTACK

Obstruction of a coronary artery or of any of its large branches has long been regarded as a serious accident. With this somber sentence James B. Herrick, M.D., began his landmark paper, in the *Journal of the American Medical Association,* December 7, 1912, on what was to become known as a heart attack. At the time of publication, other physicians had already written personal accounts of patients who had died after experiencing the crushing pain of angina pectoris —literally, "compression of the chest"—but they frequently and mistakenly attributed the cause of death to acute indigestion.

By and large, angina pectoris (or, simply, angina) was not associated with heart disease until the early decades of the 1900s when Dr. Herrick and a handful of other physicians recognized the relationship between chest pain, obstructed coronary arteries and heart damage, and published their findings from laboratory experiments and from case studies of patients. Although this was not the dawn of heart attacks—they had probably been around for millennia—it did herald the beginning of our understanding of how heart attacks occur and what they do.

As Dr. Herrick and a few others like him pointed out, an obstructed coronary artery need not be lethal. In some instances the victim could survive the attack and his heart could survive the damage. Gradually the puzzling process that begins with coronary artery disease and ends with a heart attack yielded its secrets.

One thing that made heart attacks so difficult for Dr. Herrick and his colleagues to decipher was that they could occur without any symptoms—painlessly—or with mild pain or with gripping pain. Some victims died instantly; others lingered for days and hung in the balance. There was no single way to have a heart attack. Another source of confusion was that in some people who died from a heart attack, the coronary arteries appeared clear, open and normal, while in others, the coronaries were obviously plugged with arteriosclerotic plaques and clots. There appeared to be nothing neat and tidy about the way heart attacks occur. On the groundwork laid by Dr. Herrick, succeeding generations of medical researchers and physicians assembled new theories to explain the differences in heart attacks, and they discovered new facts about how the heart works and where it goes wrong. But the cause of most heart attacks remains the same as it probably always has been: it begins in the coronary arteries.

Turbulence in the flow of blood through the coronary arteries, particularly where they branch or change direction, can damage the delicate arterial lining cells, resulting in the deposition of cholesterol from the blood. This in turn stimulates the outgrowth of muscle cells from within the media—a kind of patch to repair the injury. When the patch is no longer needed, it dissipates. But with repeated injury over the years, the patch is thought to enlarge rather than dissolve, evolving into the classical arteriosclerotic plaque composed of connective tissue, cholesterol and calcium. When such a plaque blocks off 60 to 70 percent or more of a coronary artery, the portion of the heart muscle which it supplies can become starved for oxygen, especially during exertion when the heart is called on to pump faster and harder. The oxygen-starved cells release chemical substances (enzymes) into the surrounding heart tissue, creating the chest pains and discomfort of angina pectoris.

The discomfort of angina, like the pain of a heart attack itself, produces a range of sensations with varying intensity. Some people describe it as a heaviness or pressure in the chest. Others locate it beneath the breastbone and call it a squeezing or choking sensation. Sometimes it seems to extend beyond the chest, to the neck, jaw or down the left arm. The progress of the disease that causes the pain is similarly unpredictable. Some people experience anginal pains on and off for many years and never have a heart attack.

In others, the first sensation of chest pain can signal a heart attack, with the pain intensifying and lasting longer than the ten minutes in which simple angina usually abates.

There is no simple way to distinguish between the discomfort of angina and that of an actual heart attack, except that one lasts longer. But waiting around to see if the discomfort goes away before calling for help can be lethal. The longest delay, doctors calculate, is not in getting care once you have called for it, but in deciding to make the call in the first place. The lesson is fairly simple: Do not take unnecessary chances. If you suspect that the discomfort is coming from your heart, get help, get to the nearest emergency room. As the cardiac specialist E. Grey Dimond, M.D., of the University of Missouri School of Medicine, says, "Any discomfort between the eyeballs and belly button can be a heart attack." But, he adds, "Use discretion." If you are at all uncertain, let the doctors at the hospital find out what's wrong with you. There is no need to feel embarrassed if they discover that you are not having a heart attack. Up to half the people admitted to cardiac care units (CCU) for electrocardiogram and blood tests (that detect enzymes released by damaged heart muscle) are found *not* to have had a heart attack. Some have indigestion; others have angina that does not progress into a full-blown attack.

During an anginal attack, a portion of the heart muscle suffers from a shortage of oxygen but recovers. In a heart attack, the oxygen-deprived muscle dies over a period that may be as long as six or seven days or as short as an hour. From the time a heart attack begins, no one—and no test—can predict how long it will last or how much damage it will cause. Nonetheless, treatment in the CCU can avert, or at least alleviate, the serious complications and, in some instances, even modify the course of the attack itself and help reduce the amount of heart muscle that could potentially die.

One day in the early 1960s when Bill Fix, cutting-room supervisor for a Seattle ski-clothing manufacturer, experienced his first anginal pains, most hospitals did not have cardiac care units. Mr. Fix was in his late forties at that time, an age when angina frequently begins. The pains, he recalls, came and went. In fact, they disappeared entirely after a few days, and he blamed the distress on—what else?—indigestion. He never thought to tell his doctor about the episode, for which, at the time, no one could fault him.

Nor did it occur to him to go to the local hospital—a situation that fortunately has changed for many men in their forties who are stricken by similar pains. Nowadays most hospitals are equipped with CCUs and can provide the care and diagnostic tests that are helping to save thousands of lives.

Fix's pains, however, recurred in 1978, when he was sixty-three years old. He remembers that they struck after he had a heavy meal or after he climbed the steep driveway to his home near Tacoma, overlooking Puget Sound. Although he did not know it then, his pains came whenever his heart muscle was forced to work at above idle. He was not aware of any heart problem and he had no idea that his coronary arteries were dangerously narrowed. Instead, he thought that his old indigestion trouble had arisen. His self-diagnosis was "gas pains," and he treated himself with antacid tablets. The funny thing about it, he remembers, is that they worked. After he had chewed a couple of tablets, the pain seemed to lessen, and after a few minutes of rest, it went away altogether. As he later learned, angina pains often fade during a few minutes rest, even without specific angina medication.

For Bill Fix, though, this knowledge came too late—far too late. The near-obstruction of one of his coronary arteries progressed within two months to a coronary occlusion, a complete stoppage. Perhaps a small blood clot lodged in the hair-thin opening, blocking the trickle of blood, or hemorrhage occurred within a plaque, or perhaps the narrowed, diseased artery suddenly contracted. No one knows exactly what happened to the affected coronary artery. But the end result would be the same no matter how it happened: with the blood supply cut off, a portion of his heart muscle began to die, creating an area of dead tissue, or infarct, the term from which the formal name for a heart attack—myocardial infarction —takes its root.

The hours-long process of Fix's heart attack began on an otherwise routine morning. Routine in every way except that Bill felt ill from severe pains in his chest, a fullness that during the morning he still mistakenly attributed to stomach gas. Later at work he felt so bad that he called his wife, Marjorie, at her job in Tacoma to ask her to make that long-delayed appointment with their family doctor. He never made it.

At 2:48 P.M., without warning, he fell to the cutting-room floor.

He was pale and struggling to get up when a fellow employee, Dan Gallion, one of the men who later would be credited with helping to save his life, ran up. "I started talking to him, got him to lie down," Gallion recalls. "Then he stopped breathing and started to get blue in the face." Gallion had been a lifeguard in high school and had updated his first-aid training in Vietnam. He felt for a pulse in the carotid artery at the side of Fix's throat, found none, noticed his still chest and dilated pupils. Bill Fix's heart had stopped beating, and by traditional standards he was dead.

This is the way coronary heart disease claims most of its dead —suddenly, without warning. Of the more than 650,000 people who died from coronary heart disease in 1980, over half succumbed before they reached the hospital, and usually not, as was formerly thought, because of a conventional heart attack. They die usually because the rhythm of the heart is disrupted and degenerates into a formless, ineffective quivering. If this life-threatening arr- hythmia, known as ventricular fibrillation, is not quickly reversed, it can progress to cardiac arrest, a term that is synonymous with no heartbeat, no pulse and zero blood pressure.

Fortunately, Dan Gallion did not give up. Trained in the tech- nique known as cardiopulmonary resuscitation (CPR), Gallion tilted Fix's head back to provide a clear air passage past the tongue, then he began breathing air into the supervisor's mouth, inflating his lungs. At that instant, manufacturing manager Dev Shaunak broke through the knot of frightened bystanders, knelt down and began the cardiac compression part of CPR, manually depressing Fix's lower breastbone strongly, rhythmically, a second a beat, to force blood through the heart and lungs and out to the body. On every fifth beat, Gallion filled Fix's lungs with his own breath. Together they knew they could keep Fix's blood circulating until help arrived, but their efforts had to be kept up steadily. Without oxygen brought by the blood, Fix's fragile brain cells would begin to die in just four minutes, his heart muscle in ten. Gratefully, Gallion noted color returning to Fix's skin—their efforts were succeeding.

Somebody had called 911—Seattle's (and many other cities') universal "help" number—and three minutes afterward, a couple of young firemen carrying rescue equipment dashed into the cut- ting room to relieve Gallion and Shaunak of their CPR duties. Not missing a beat, they continued the chest compression but substituted an air-bag bellows for the mouth-to-mouth breathing. Two minutes later a more highly trained pair of fire-department rescuers rushed in and set to work on the prostrate Fix. Paramedics Michael Foley and Barry Newcomb slapped two metal paddles against Fix's chest, took an electrocardiographic reading which confirmed that the heart rhythm was ventricular fibrillation, then shocked it back into a regular rhythm with a single jolt of electricity. Consulting by radio with a doctor back at their base at Harborview Medical Center, they injected a drug to combat further fibrillation, inserted an intravenous tube to infuse still other drugs, and passed a breathing tube down into his lungs, attaching it to a mechanical pump that breathed for him. When Fix seemed out of immediate danger, the paramedics transported him in their ambulance to the cardiac care unit at Harborview, where he began his recovery from the puzzling condition doctors refer to simply as "sudden death."

Bill Fix represents a new kind of patient in American hospitals, never before seen because all formerly died. The number of such "revived dead" will grow as more cities like Cleveland, Dallas, Houston, St. Paul, Miami, Jacksonville, Dayton and Washington, D.C., follow Seattle's lead in developing sophisticated rescue systems backed up by a citizenry trained in CPR. The last is vital. In Seattle—a city justifiably world-famous for its rapid-response emergency care system—where one resident in five has been trained in CPR, 43 percent of sudden-death patients who received bystander-initiated CPR survived to be discharged from the hospital. When bystanders did not initiate CPR, but waited for the fire-department rescuers, only 21 percent of patients survived. Potentially, says Leonard A. Cobb, M.D., chief of cardiology at Harborview Medical Center and founder and director of the Seattle Fire Department's emergency medical care system, two thirds of sudden death victims could be saved by immediate resuscitation. This optimism confirms the wisdom of the famous heart surgeon Claude Beck that these hearts are "too good to die."

There are two broad types of heart attack: the standard model, which doctors call a myocardial infarction (MI), and the sudden-death version. Bill Fix had both.

MIs come in all shapes and sizes and produce a variety of symptoms. A San Francisco sheet-metal worker recalls that his heart attack felt "like somebody was stomping on my chest." A distinguished cardiologist experienced all the classic symptoms: a sickening, heavy, aching sensation beneath his breastbone (not the temporary pains of angina, which he had experienced before, but lasting for hours), the pain radiating to his jaw and down his left arm, with breathlessness, sweating and nausea. And then there are people who did not even know they had a heart attack. Electrocardiograph screening of middle-aged men consistently turns up evidence of "silent heart attacks"—perhaps painless, perhaps passed off as indigestion. Still other attacks are preceded by days or weeks of bone-tired fatigue.

A heart attack that affects a small but vital area of the heart—an area called the sinoatrial node, which initiates and paces beat—can be far more dangerous than an attack that destroys a larger amount of muscle but spares the conduction pathways. Damaged heart-muscle cells, deprived of oxygen during an attack that is triggered by a blockage in a coronary artery, release small electrical impulses that may deflect and disrupt that heart's normal electrical signals, emanating from its internal pacemaker. These are the ways the standard model heart attack can turn into ventricular fibrillation, the sudden-death version that struck down Bill Fix. Fortunately, however, most people who have the standard model heart attack do not develop ventricular fibrillation because the damage spares the sinoatrial tissue and the conduction pathway between the ventricles. Nevertheless, a massive heart attack can destroy so much heart muscle that the pumping ability of the left ventricle is impaired beyond its capacity to support life.

About 15 to 20 percent of ventricular-fibrillation incidents occur —as in Bill Fix's case—as the result of an ongoing MI. Most of the rest are the result of previous damage from MIs. The consensus among cardiologists is that MIs make the heart more vulnerable to fibrillation. "About forty percent of our sudden-death patients," Harborview's Dr. Cobb says, "have a history of MI, and another fifteen to twenty percent have had a heart attack and don't know it, but there is evidence of heart muscle damage on their electrocardiograms." For still largely unknown reasons, a heart that has been damaged by coronary artery disease can suddenly go into fibrillation. It can happen anytime and anywhere, but it is more likely to happen during a heart attack and during the recovery period. This is why getting help quickly is so important.

Why does ventricular fibrillation occur at a particular moment? Very possibly the nervous system has something to do with it. Cardiologists also theorize that an imbalance in the system of minerals known as electrolytes, especially potassium, upon which the heart's electrical action depends, can trigger the useless quivering of ventricular fibrillation. Regardless of how it happened to Bill Fix, he was saved, but not before he had the attention and specialized care of a number of people—the cardiac care and rehabilitation team assembled from many departments at Seattle's Harborview Medical Center, a hospital not unlike hundreds of others throughout the United States that have drawn upon their own resourcefulness and the expertise of their staff to bring heart-attack victims back to life, and equally as important, back to the enjoyment of living without the crushing fear that disabled so many heart-attack patients not all that long ago.

Day One

Bill Fix lay unconscious in Harborview's CCU, his arms strung with tubes and wires, his mouth and nose covered by a respirator mask, his chest moving up and down to the rhythm of the mechanical ventilator. Electrical signals from his heart were picked up by electrodes attached to his chest and limbs, and they were displayed on the fluorescent screen of an oscilloscope next to his bed. An audible tone—*beep-beep-beep*—kept pace with the electrical projection of his heartbeat as the bright dot of light made its jagged path across the screen. This monitor would sound an alarm if the heart rhythm changed for the worse. Irregular beats, or arrhythmias, are common during the first twenty-four to forty-eight hours following a heart attack, and before the days of coronary care units, such irregularities often were not caught or reversed in time.

One of the bottles, hanging from an IV stand above the bed, silently dripped a solution of lidocaine down a clear plastic tube inserted into one of Bill's arms. The fluid has a quieting effect on the heart, steadying its beat. If an arrhythmia occurred, despite the lidocaine, a more powerful antiarrhythmic agent was immediately available and could be injected within seconds. Or in the event of ventricular fibrillation, an electric defibrillator (a device that discharges very brief bursts of direct-current electricity across the chest and into the heart muscle in order to stop arrhythmia) was nearby to shock the heart back to its regular beat, as had been done by the paramedics who brought Fix to the hospital. By such measures, together with frequent monitoring of blood chemistry, intake and outgo of fluids, and by administering various medications, hospital deaths from heart attacks have been cut in the last twenty years from 30 to 35 percent to 10 to 15 percent. (Another reason for the drop in mortality, according to Dr. Cobb, is that people are learning to minimize and eliminate their heart-disease risk factors and, therefore, "we may be seeing milder cases today.")

Outside the CCU, before she saw her husband, Marjorie Fix was consoled and counseled by a social worker who briefly described what to expect, but nothing could fully prepare her for this experience. A few hours before, as both she and Bill headed for work, she had said goodbye to a smiling, apparently healthy husband. Now he was gravely ill, and the elaborateness of the equipment around his bed only emphasized the dramatic measures that were being taken to save him. The predicament her husband was in was mirrored on Marjorie's face as she stood over him; the CCU nurse recognized this and was ready to help.

Reassurance is not only important to the patient, once recovery begins, but also to the patient's family, starting from the time treatment begins. But like the medical attention itself, psychological reassurance is a "one day at a time" process. The questions patients and their families ask take days and even weeks to be fully answered, and their equally important fears require untold hours of understanding on everyone's part to be resolved. Nonetheless, the process began the moment Marjorie looked up at the nurse.

She had spoken to her husband, hoping that he would awaken from his coma, but when there was no response, the nurse knew that the first of many questions was on its way. His unconsciousness, she explained, resulted from the fact that his brain was temporarily injured from lack of oxygen during the sudden-death episode. It was swollen and pressed against the confining vault of the skull. No one could say with certainty when he might open his eyes, and even when he did, there would be days of confusion ahead. In the meantime, she said, "he is in the best of hands," but the words seemed to float in the air as Marjorie allowed herself the emotional release of tears. The comfort of a touch by her husband's nurse was the first bridge of trust that would be extended in the days to come.

Day Two

The charts showed that the patient passed an "uneventful night." Later that morning, with Fix still unconscious, one of the CCU doctors injected a local anesthetic into his arm and threaded a thin plastic tube, with a tiny balloon and sensing devices in its tip (known as a Swan-Ganz catheter) through an arm vein into the right atrium of the heart, down to the right ventricle, and finally into one of the pulmonary arteries leading to the lungs. The balloon was inflated to lodge it firmly in the vessel, and the sensors began monitoring the blood pressure on both sides of the balloon, measuring, in effect, the pressure of the left atrium. The pressure reading transmitted from one side of the balloon showed the pumping force of the heart's right ventricle, the reading from the other side registered back pressure from the left atrium and left ventricle. Fix's reading was slightly elevated. A higher reading could have indicated that his heart was failing, as a result of the heart attack having damaged a large percentage of the muscle, and could no longer pump strongly enough to meet the body's demands for oxygen. Then the doctors would have used a specific vasodilator drug to open up the arterioles (tiny arteries throughout the body through which blood passes from larger arteries to the capillaries) to decrease resistance and ease the burden on the heart and to relax the veins, reducing the amount of blood returning to the heart.

As it was, Fix's heart was not failing, and near noon, shortly after the respirator was removed, he began to regain consciousness. Nurses removed the remaining catheters and wires and moved Fix to an "intermediate care" room nearby, but still within the CCU and open on the corridor side so that he was always in full view from the nurses' station. For most heart-attack patients at Harborview, this move happens on the second or third day, on the proven theory that they are largely out of danger after the first twenty-four to forty-eight hours.

The remaining electrodes taped to Fix's chest were attached to a small radio transmitter, and this, in turn, was strapped to his waist, making it possible for him to move about freely while the electrical signals of his heartbeat were still transmitted to a monitor in his room and to a console at the nurses' station. This would become especially useful later when the nurses walked him down the hall or he attempted a new exercise. The monitors would show how much activity he could handle—no guesswork about it. If any activity caused an arrhythmia or if he experienced angina pain, it was stopped immediately.

During all this activity, which was actually accomplished calmly and unhurriedly over the remainder of the afternoon, Fix learned what had happened to him and where he was, then promptly forgot and asked the same questions again. His mind reverted back twelve years—like being in a time machine, he later explained. When asked where he lived, he gave the address and telephone number of the house from which he and Marjorie had moved ten years earlier. He spoke of weekending at "the cottage on the Sound near Tacoma"—for many years now their permanent home—and of just speaking with friends in the old neighborhood, people he had not seen in a decade. The Fix's nineteen-year old daughter, Linda, just starting her second year of college in Bellingham, Washington, had rushed back home to be with her father, who remembered her only as a seven-year-old. After a pleasant chat he startled his daughter by asking, "Where's your dad?"

Brain damage is the dark side of the CPR picture. In relatively few instances this can mean permanent mental deficiencies or permanent coma. The longer it takes to begin resuscitation, the greater the possibility of brain cells dying. Over half of the sudden-death victims resuscitated solely by Seattle paramedics—who have to travel to the victim, thus using up precious time—suffer major neurologic deficit when discharged from the hospital. In time, most of them recover completely, as Bill Fix did. But only 4 percent of those resuscitated by the quick action of people on the scene have such a deficit when they are sent home from the hospital.

If sudden death had been Bill Fix's only problem, he might have been on his way to going home. Usually sudden-death victims suffer no obvious heart damage and are not treated like regular heart patients. If they experience no arrhythmias for forty-eight hours, they can soon go home and return to work, but they must continue taking antiarrhythmic medication. Such patients also usually have coronary arteriograms (chest x-rays taken after the injection of a dye into the bloodstream which show the coronary arteries) to determine whether they are candidates for bypass surgery.

Day Three

Although an electrocardiogram taken on the day Fix was admitted showed an abnormal pattern indicative of a heart attack, it could not reveal when it had occurred—a day, a week or years before. Hypothetically, in a court of law, this might be called presumptive evidence that a heart attack actually precipitated his ventricular fibrillation. But in a hospital, doctors have a definitive way of telling when—and if—a heart attack occurred by analyzing the blood over three days for the presence of various enzymes produced in increased quantities by the body when heart tissue dies. Specific enzymes that are measured in the days immediately after a heart attack are serum glutamic oxaloacetic transaminase (SGOT), creatine phosphokinase (CPK) and lactic dehydrogenase (LDH).

Fix's three-day enzyme pattern, peaking on the second day, showed that he had suffered a mild heart attack on the day he was admitted. To assess the functioning of his heart and the extent of the damage, Fix underwent a battery of diagnostic tests beginning with x-rays of his chest to determine whether or not his heart was enlarged. It was not, but if it had been, doctors would have had another indication of impending heart failure. An enlarged heart, following a heart attack, is an indication that the main pumping chambers—the left and right ventricles—are unable to pump out all the blood that is delivered to them because too much muscle has been damaged. Thus, one or both ventricles engorges with excess blood, and this shows up on the x-ray as an enlarged heart. Next, a harmless, mildly radioactive tracer was injected into his bloodstream. The tracer is absorbed by healthy heart muscle, but not by damaged or dead muscle. Specialized equipment, partly resembling a TV screen, is able to pick up the tracer and produce an image of the heart that appears white where it is healthy and black where it is not. The tracer test showed that Fix's heart-attack damage was not extensive, perhaps no more than an inch or two across, and that it probably did not extend completely through the left ventricular wall.

Heart attacks most frequently damage the left ventricle—as Fix's did—because the coronary artery that feeds this chamber is the one most frequently affected by arteriosclerosis. Had Fix suffered a severe heart attack, and had the damage been large—with 40 percent or more of his left ventricle destroyed—he probably would not have survived despite the successful effort to restore an effective heart rhythm through electrical conversion of the fibrillation. Other images would be taken on successive days to determine if the darkened area decreased in size, indicating that not all of the damage from the attack was permanent.

To characterize the heart function, Fix was also given an echocardiogram, a test that shoots harmless sound waves into the chest and captures their echoes, which are transformed into a moving picture of the heart on a TV screen. The picture clearly displays movements of the walls and valves of the heart, and distortions caused by noncontracting dead or injured heart muscle. Evidence from this test supported the findings from the tracer test—namely, that the left ventricle had a small abnormality in its movement centered in the area where an artery was clogged and heart tissue had died.

The irregular heartbeats which follow almost all heart attacks had been under control for nearly twelve hours by the afternoon of the third day, and Bill was deemed well enough to be moved out of the CCU into a standard hospital room without special heart-monitoring equipment. For some patients, this move is traumatic. They come to depend for their lives on the robot "guardian angel" monitoring their every heartbeat. But Bill took the move in his stride. Once he was settled in, he was told, another electronic watchdog, known as a Holter monitor, would take the place of the larger bedside device. The Holter monitor is a miniature electrocardiograph that continuously records the heartbeat for twenty-four hours or longer on a cassette tape, which can be played back in a computer-assisted reader, enabling the patient's doctors to view a speeded-up daily record of the heart waves in a few minutes, or to stop and "freeze" tracings at will, or to examine only those intervals in which the ECG tracing is abnormal. Fix was asked to keep a careful record of his activities for the time he was wearing the Holter monitor—noting when he took medicine or a nap or when he had a meal or walked down the hall —so that his doctors could analyze the function of Fix's heart, and adjust his regimen accordingly.

Day Four and Onward

As Bill Fix's normal alertness returned, he became an active partner in his recovery, asking questions about the nature of his disease and about the adjustment in lifestyle that he would have to make. The major change for him would be giving up cigarettes after forty-five years of smoking. He was already watching his diet, so that would not be a problem, and since he had normal blood pressure, he would not have to restrict his salt intake. These initial questions about diet arose because he, like other heart patients at Harborview, subsisted on a 1,200-calorie a day diet (liquid the first day) that is designed to spare the heart from extra work during digestion, and Fix had asked about it. Although a certain amount of exercise is important to keep the blood from getting sluggish and possibly forming a clot, the heart needs rest while it heals, and the less strain put on it by digestion, he was told, the better. Thus the light diet.

In the first stages of the healing process, which had already begun in Fix's heart, white blood corpuscles enter the damaged heart muscle and remove the dead heart cells, and scar tissue gradually forms to seal the wound. This tough, fibrous replacement tissue does not contract like normal heart muscle, thus it does no work, and at times it might even interfere with the electrical signals from the heart's natural pacemaker and cause an arrhythmia. But it is as strong or stronger than the muscle it replaces and it is insensitive to pain, so it will not cause angina.

The healing process typically takes from three to six weeks, which is why, only a generation ago, heart patients remained in the hospital six weeks. According to Bert Green, M.D., director of cardiac rehabilitation at Seattle's University Hospital, "Doctors, at the time, were afraid the heart would rupture if it were strained before it had a chance to heal. But now there are powerful arguments against lying in bed immobilized for a month or longer. Lengthy bed rest increases the risk of pulmonary embolism [a blood clot that forms in the leg veins and travels to the lungs], besides weakening the body's muscles from the inactivity. With weakened muscles, the patient, once at home, finds physical effort harder than before, more taxing on the heart. And so today the trend is to get heart patients out of bed sooner and get them home earlier."

By the early 1970s the standard hospital stay had been reduced to three weeks of bed rest combined with moderate exercise. Now it is two weeks, and in some uncomplicated cases, less. Modern cardiac rehabilitation, though, is not limited to the physical side of the patient. It has expanded to include the emotional, psychological, social, vocational and practical aspects of the person's life as well, and had Bill Fix known that he was being "rehabilitated" in half a dozen different ways, he might have resisted the program to remold him. Yet it came at him subtly and reasonably. In fact, cardiac rehabilitation is often a natural response to the patient's own concerns.

The nurses and social workers who stopped by to see Fix encouraged this natural inclination to ask questions. In one conversation, Fix began wondering aloud whether or not stress caused his attack. There were always problems at work, he said, production snags, rush orders, but he could not see giving up a job he genuinely liked and did so well. Then, on his own initiative, the subject of whether and when he could go back to work was broached for the first time and he was invited to listen to a variety of tape-recorded rehabilitation lectures, on topics ranging from symptoms, to what to look for after discharge, to sexual activity.

One of the fears—if not the major one—after a heart attack is the fear of dying. Kim Clark, the Harborview social worker who was assigned to coronary care during Bill Fix's stay, said that all the heart-attack patients she has seen believed that they were going to die, and Bill was no different. Once he began talking about this fear, she said, it opened the floodgates to others. His willingness to talk about his feelings was viewed as a healthy sign that he was beginning to deal with the problems that invariably arise in the aftermath of a heart attack—problems that revolve around loss of health, money (medical and hospital bills), loss of the strong husband-provider role, and loss of control.

The ramifications of these problems extend beyond the patient, and as so often happens, it is the spouse who is faced with new —and potentially frightening—responsibilities. For months after a heart-attack patient returns home, perhaps forever, husband and wife must function in new roles. In making the adjustment, certain problems and questions are bound to occur. Some of the most frequent sources of concern follow:

Mood Problems

It is natural for a wife to experience some amount of panic just before her husband is discharged or for a husband to experience the same feelings if his wife has had a heart attack. To smooth the transition from hospital to home, it is a good idea to talk about the tasks that lie ahead, to iron out the rough spots about who will take care of what and to anticipate as much as possible how the day-to-day responsibilities will be divided. People who have recovered from a heart attack admit that it is degrading to lie in bed and have everything done for them. But on the other hand, their spouses are afraid that if they don't "do everything," another heart attack could occur. One partner is depressed, the other is scared—and there is nothing unnatural about these feelings. They happen, and it is important to admit what is going on, not to hide it. Ultimately, the responsibility for getting on with living rests with the person who has suffered the heart attack. Emotional support can only go so far, and before it runs out, both parties are liable to feel angry. In fact, anger in a recovering heart patient is as normal as depression. Strange as it may seem, the person who has had the heart attack and the person who is changing the sheets and cooking the meals can both feel sorry and angry at the same time. Sorry for what has happened and angry that it has happened to them. That is not meant to encourage shouting matches—which can strain the heart in more ways than one. But admitting the anger, talking about it, is one way to clear the air.

Sex Problems

Sex after a heart attack is a great source of unnecessary fear for both husband and wife. Some heart patients fear that sex will precipitate another heart attack. The patient's spouse may feel even more apprehensive; if something happens, the guilt would be hard to bear. But according to studies on this subject, the typical marital sexual encounter is no more taxing than climbing two flights of stairs, and individual physicians usually counsel both husband and wife on the appropriate timing for resumption of sexual activity. Restrictions vary depending upon heart damage and general health. If the husband is the one who had the heart attack, he may be instructed to assume the passive role during intercourse for the first few weeks. If sex brings on angina, it may be possible to prevent the pains with nitroglycerin tablets ahead of time. Regular exercise, such as walking, bicycling or jogging can improve a patient's stamina and help prevent anginal pains during sexual activity.

Children Problems

The time after a parent comes home can be one of great togetherness, usually beneficial rather than difficult for the children. Children are often delighted to take care of a parent; it makes them feel important, and doing something for the parent helps to relieve their worries. One note of caution: do not let a child assume most of the responsibility for the care of a parent; if something should go wrong—onset of another heart attack, for example—the child might bear too much guilt.

Singles' Problems

If there is no one to come home to, there are extra difficulties. Waiting for her husband to be wheeled back from a laboratory procedure, Marjorie Fix fell into conversation with an elderly retired businesswoman who was about to be discharged. Never married, the woman lived alone with her cat in a well-kept high-rise apartment and had always been proud of her self-sufficiency.

She had no relatives living in Seattle, and few close friends, and she barely knew her neighbors. She wondered how she would shop for groceries, make a bed, wash clothes or prepare a meal during the next few days. She felt weak and was supposed to remain quiet.

The dilemma, Marjorie Fix later learned, brought out the retired woman's resourcefulness. It forced her to reach out to other people. For soft-drink and movie money, her neighbor's teen-age daughter promised to help out with household chores for an hour each day after school. The janitor's son went shopping for her. Restricted from going out evenings, she got on the phone and invited acquaintances to stop by, which they did.

These same problems are not so easily solved for every heart-attack patient who is single. Some are already disabled from arthritis, diabetes or other ailments and were barely able to make it alone before the attack. Almost any hospital, through its social-service department, will help a homebound patient locate a homemaker to assume household duties and a visiting nurse to attend to personal care.

Money Problems

Finances frequently add to the burden of a heart attack. At the time Bill Fix was hospitalized, in 1978, CCU expenses were upwards of $500 a day. The bill from the physicians who treated him was $735, and his hospital charges totaled $7,365, almost 50 percent more than the average for a heart attack treated at Harborview because his stay was longer than average. Fortunately, like many other employed people, the Fixes were covered with comprehensive health insurance through their employers. Bill's policy covered all his doctors' bills plus 80 percent of the hospital bill, a total of $6,732. And Marjorie's family policy absorbed all but a few dollars of the remainder.

A middle-aged salesman who shared a room with Fix for a few days was less fortunate. The bill for his heart-attack care was not over $5,000, but he was unemployed and carried no health insurance. His fretting was relieved after a social worker suggested that he might be eligible for Medicaid. He had not thought of applying for it, even though he had no savings to speak of, because he owned his own home and assumed that any property made him ineligible. Ultimately, Medicaid paid his entire hospital and medical bill. He was not forced to sell his house; one's residence is specifically exempted from calculations in figuring Medicaid eligibility. He was also allowed to keep his car, which the government considers essential in order to look for work and keep a job.

Another patient Bill Fix met was only partially covered by his health insurance. The hospital arranged for a time-payment plan beginning only after he returned to his job.

Eventually the time for discharge comes, and all the information imparted during informal chats, counseling sessions, rehabilitation lectures and doctor-patient discussion has to be translated into the practicalities of everyday life. For Fix, this came on his discharge day. He still felt bruised from his Lazarus experience. His ribs ached from the resuscitation efforts—as they would for some six months—and he had little stamina. But these were trifles, for he was going home.

His medication routine had been ironed out during his stay, and he was given written instructions for the pills he needed to take every day. Although he had no further problems with irregular beats, he was advised to wear the Holter monitor at home on different occasions, twenty-four hours at a time, so that his cardiologist would have a record of his heart-wave pattern as Fix's heart continued to strengthen.

Bill experienced little of the boredom and frustration that send many recuperating heart patients up the proverbial wall. He loved to read, and he passed many days absorbed in a novel or biography. When his eyes tired, he refreshed them by gazing out his picture window upon the ever-changing waters of Puget Sound and the sky above, and beyond to the snow-clad Olympic range piercing the western horizon. He was, by all accounts, glad to be alive, and rightly so, after his close brush with death.

Unlike many male heart patients, he did not resent the fact that he now stayed home while his wife went to work. After so many years as a breadwinner, his role was not threatened by the temporary change, because he had been assured that his old job would be waiting for him when he felt ready to take over the supervisory reins again.

At first Marjorie Fix was concerned about continuing to live in their home, which, at eight miles from the nearest sizable town, she felt was too far from emergency help in case of another cardiac arrest. But she solved her own worries without moving by organizing CPR classes at her office, and she enrolled in the first class taught by a Red Cross paramedic. If necessary, she hoped, she would be able to revive her husband and keep him alive until help arrived. (For help in finding where such CPR courses are given, contact your local Red Cross or the chapter of the American Heart Association in your area.)

Bill's cardiologist had advised walking as the best exercise prescription to strengthen muscles weakened by bed rest and to improve his general health. As his endurance improved, he broadened this into a do-it-yourself exercise program. Yet had he and his doctor preferred, he could have taken a different approach that is increasingly popular. In Seattle—as in Cleveland, New York, Boston, Miami, Milwaukee, Kansas City, Chicago, Washington, D.C., and scores of other cities—doctors refer recent victims of heart attacks to organized exercise programs especially designed for heart patients, where the individual's performance on a treadmill or bicycle ergometer is evaluated and an exercise prescription is designed to strengthen his heart. (For a list of qualified places that offer supervised exercise programs for heart patients, either consult your own physician or call your local chapter of the American Heart Association.)

The alternative to not exercising can turn a heart-attack victim into what has been labeled a "cardiac cripple"—a person who might have been told to get some exercise but not to overdo it, and is then afraid, in the extreme, to even walk from the car to his house. A sixty-five-year-old minister was well on his way to getting this opprobrious label after returning home from his heart attack. He lay in bed nearly all day, scared of what any activity would do to his heart, even though he had been advised to exercise for an hour each day. Three months after his heart attack, when he was still ignoring his doctor's advice to get out and walk around, he was referred to CAPRI, Seattle's Cardio-Pulmonary Research Institute, where he was given an exercise stress test to determine the outside limits of his endurance, and then was enrolled in an exercise class. At first he could barely walk the prescribed number of laps around the gymnasium, but soon he was jogging a bit, alternating with walking, and he began to look forward to the camaraderie of the thrice-weekly training sessions. Two and a half years later, on the exercise stress test, he scored at 116 percent of the norm for men his age. "I'm feeling better, looking better, and even my sermons are better," he said.

Another CAPRI participant tells of an unsuccessful heart operation a decade ago. Her physician scheduled her for a second operation, but sent her first to CAPRI to get her in better shape for surgery. The training, she says, made the second operation unnecessary. Perhaps the most dramatic story, though, is that of a sixty-one-year-old man who had experienced two heart attacks, suffered terribly from angina and had a very bad electrocardiogram. Since he couldn't even walk around the gym once without turning blue, someone rigged up an oxygen tank on a golf cart so that he could whiff oxygen from a hose as he ambled around the circular track. Within a year he was jogging one mile a session, and his angina had disappeared. No one can prove that a cardiac exercise program reduces heart attacks or extends life, but it definitely enhanced the lives of these and thousands of other participants.

With the support of his wife, Bill Fix reaped the same satisfaction from exercise, and the same benefit, on his own. After a few months he was back at work part-time, and soon thereafter full-time. He is "different" only in the sense that a certain time is missing from his life. He cannot recall anything about the day he dropped dead or the week following. He knows only what he has been told about this critical period, and that he owes his life to modern coronary care.

In 1981 approximately 800,000 Americans suffered their first heart attacks, and of these about 350,000 died. They did not have the opportunity that Bill Fix did to recover and change their risk factors. They did not get that second chance.

Thousands of people, though, do get a second chance. The statistics prove it. But what they do not often show is that about 600,000 people a year suffer a second or third or fourth heart attack, and about half of them die.

These two groups—those succumbing to their first attacks and those dying after a second or subsequent attack—account for the 650,000 deaths from heart attacks in 1981.

Survival of a heart attack is no free ticket to a long life. Risk factors need to be modified, drugs sometimes have to be taken, surgery is indicated at times. Nonetheless, in concert with those who care about you and with your physicians, and with your best interests in mind, you can keep on living.

The risk of having a second heart attack can be sharply reduced. The evidence comes from two landmark studies on drugs that have been used in the United States since 1966, but for purposes other than that of preventing a second heart attack.

The drugs are beta-blockers, and they are used to control high blood pressure, treat angina and stop abnormal heart rhythms.

A Norwegian study on the beta-blocker called timolol maleate showed that the chance of suffering a second heart attack or dying of a sudden rhythm abnormality is significantly reduced for up to seventeen months after a heart attack.

A study on a similar beta-blocker called propranolol hydrochloride was cut short by its sponsor, the National Heart, Lung and Blood Institute, because the results were so overwhelmingly favorable that the investigators realized they could not deny beta-blocker treatment to the control group. The death rate was reduced by 26 percent among heart attack victims who took propranolol in an effort to prevent another attack. William T. Friedewald, M.D., associate director for clinical applications and prevention at the Heart, Lung and Blood Institute, said that the results of the Beta-Blocker Heart Attack Trial have implications for the 350,000 Americans who are discharged from hospitals each year following their first heart attacks. About two thirds, and perhaps as many as three fourths, are eligible for beta-blocker therapy.

It is estimated that beta-blockers may be able to save thousands of lives a year in the United States by thwarting a second heart attack.

The way these drugs protect the heart in people who have had a heart attack is not yet fully understood, but there is some evidence that they reduce the risk of serious ventricular rhythm disturbances. The drugs received their name because they block the beta receptor sites that are found on cells throughout the body. These sites in heart muscle cells are sensitive to adrenalin. When the levels of adrenalin increase in the bloodstream or when adrenalin is directed to the heart's beta receptors, the heart muscle responds by speeding up its beat.

Should adrenalin be prevented from getting to the beta receptors, the heart muscle will either slow its rate of contraction or simply not respond to the stimulation in the first place. In essence, this is what happens with beta-blocker medication.

For people like Bill Fix who have had a heart attack, beta-blockers can be a lifesaver. These drugs, and some others described in later chapters, are revolutionizing the treatment of people with heart disease.

13

CARDIAC ARREST

A generation ago, while investigating how the heart and the rest of the body's internal systems respond to external emergencies, the renowned Harvard physiology professor Walter B. Cannon, M.D., became intrigued by reports of "death spells" that explorers had witnessed in their travels among primitive peoples in Africa, Haiti, Brazil and the South Pacific. Could a dark and forbidding ritual that is infused with the power of suggestion literally kill its intended victim? And if so, how?

Drawn by his curiosity about the human mind and its influence on internal organs, Dr. Cannon began his methodical and scientific probe into the phenomenon of voodoo death. His studies confirmed beyond a doubt that a spell cast by a voodoo priest could cause death, and he went on to show that the underlying mechanism was not a hidden poison or anything else tangible. It was fear. The psychological fright of being marked for death, of having no one to turn to (because the ritual spell strips all social support from the victim), can cause vast and irreparable physiological damage that Dr. Cannon found could actually cause the victim to die suddenly.

At the time, this excursion into the phenomenon of voodoo was only a waystation along the route to other theories that Dr. Cannon was developing and testing—theories that would establish his name in the annals of medical history. He became widely known for describing the "flight or fight" reaction, the physiological response to emergency situations that begins with the release of adrenalin into the bloodstream. And he laid the groundwork for the theories that implicate stress as a primary factor in the cause of many diseases. Dr. Cannon's ideas about the power of suggestion and his notions about voodoo spells emerged decades after his death as one in a series of clues that has given medical science a new understanding of the heart and its relationship to the brain.

Another important piece of evidence in this relationship came from George Engel, M.D., who reported on the seemingly unusual circumstances surrounding several deaths that had come to his attention at the Rochester University Medical School. One involved a fifty-five-year-old man who was to be united with his eighty-eight-year-old father after a twenty-year separation. At the meeting the son keeled over, an apparent victim of sudden death. A few seconds later the same fate befell the father. Other cases involved a husband and wife who died of heart attacks within thirteen hours of each other, and a father who dropped dead while comforting a son who had just been injured in a motorcycle accident.

There were even disquieting reports of the frightening effect that doctors sometimes have on patients. In one hospital, for instance, sudden death was five times as likely to occur during daily medical rounds as at any other time. Could these instances of overwhelming emotion and sudden death be the modern equivalent of Cannon's tenet linking mortal fear and voodoo death? That thought occurred to Bernard Lown, M.D., now a professor of cardiology at Harvard Medical School and a world authority on arrhythmias and the sudden death they often produce.

In 1960 Dr. Lown became fascinated by the link between the mind and what was once thought to be the seat of the soul—the heart. In the years since then, he has come to believe that one's thoughts and feelings can help protect one's own heart. Although he and his associates at Harvard's Cardiovascular Laboratories analyze and treat dangerous rhythms of the heart with a wide spectrum of drugs and the most sophisticated technical equipment, they are finding that the ultimate instrument to treat arrhythmias and prevent sudden death may be the human mind itself.

This may sound heretical, but the weight of the evidence says it is not. And even though some of the techniques and principles Dr.

Lown and his colleagues have pioneered are controversial, they are being used in conjunction with conventional therapy and medication to reduce the toll of sudden death. Two decades ago, when Dr. Lown began investigating the arrhythmias that led up to sudden death, ventricular fibrillation was the leading cause of death in the United States, claiming 400,000 to 450,000 lives annually—1,200 a day, or nearly one a minute. That terrible pace has not slackened, but inroads are being made, thanks to Dr. Lown and others, into the cause, treatment and prevention of sudden death.

Only in rare circumstances is the normal heart in danger of ventricular fibrillation. Between 75 and 90 percent of the people who suffer this sudden, ineffective rhythm, according to Dr. Lown, have coronary artery disease. Not all of them have heart-attack damage during a sudden-death episode. Many, in fact, have never suffered a heart attack, nor are they aware beforehand that anything is amiss within their hearts. Nevertheless, there is reason, Dr. Lown believes, to suspect that portions of their hearts were temporarily starved for oxygen due to a clog or a spasm in a coronary artery when ventricular fibrillation occurred.

"The tragic thing about sudden death from my point of view, and what impelled me to study it," Dr. Lown says, "was the fact that it doesn't come at the end of life where it can be a blessing. It interrupts life almost at its apogee—it strikes down people at the average age of fifty-nine or sixty. It is more common in men than women. If you visit the retirement havens of our country, in Florida, California or Arizona, you'll see mostly widows. Where are the men? They dropped dead. The fact that the life expectancy of women is six to eight years greater than men can be laid to this one cause—sudden cardiac death."

Before the 1960s, Dr. Lown says, "doctors remained somewhat indifferent to the problem for a number of reasons. In the first place, it seemed like an act of God. Secondly, it occurred outside the doctor's purview—in the community, before the victim could reach a hospital. Thirdly, the doctor had the preconception that sudden death was the culmination of far advanced and inexorably advancing atherosclerosis, and therefore was nigh irreversible."

Then, in the mid-1960s, doctors discovered a way to restore a fibrillating heart to normal rhythm by means of an electric current applied to the chest. Thousands of heart patients prone to arrhythmias came under surveillance in the newly developed coronary care units. Astonishingly, some victims of sudden death could be revived and live. What struck Dr. Lown as so unusual at the time was that he expected them to go ahead and die again in the next minute or so. But they did not. They lived—for a year, two years and more. It did not make sense to him, and the only conclusion he could draw was that sudden death is an electrical accident—an accident that extinguishes life but is reversible. His work soon focused on two questions: first, How do you protect the heart? and second, Why does sudden death occur at the moment it does?

Step by step his research group built a case to prove that increased neural activity—thoughts and feelings—can provoke irregularities in the heart's rhythm that may degenerate into the chaotic, disorganized beating that leads to sudden death. In laboratory experiments, dogs whose hearts previously had been damaged from myocardial infarction were conditioned to expect an electric shock when they were placed in a fearful setting. The research showed that it took 50 percent less energy (delivered directly to the heart muscle, and not felt by the animal) to produce ventricular fibrillation in these dogs than when they were in a nonfearful setting.

Data gathered from electrocardiograms on hospitalized patients also had shown that a certain type of rhythm disturbance, known as premature ventricular contraction—sometimes felt as a skipped beat, and not harmful in the normal heart—indicated risk for sudden death in persons with heart disease. Doctors believe that these premature contractions are somehow related to inadequate blood flow to the heart muscle. When the heart is forced to work hard, as it is during stress, these telltale blips may start appearing on the electrocardiograph. The next logical research step was to find out whether these premature beats could be triggered in people who are in mentally stressful situations.

In a now classic experiment, Dr. Lown's group found that they could. Nineteen people were given confusing mental arithmetic problems and then were urged to talk about their fears regarding death, money and marital problems. During this psychological stress test, some of the participants' pulse rate doubled on the average, and premature ventricular beats started appearing on the electrocardiograph. Based on this and similar research, Dr. Lown and many other cardiologists now try to provoke arrhythmias under controlled circumstances in patients with known heart disease, using either a mental or a physical stress test. In this way they are able to identify patients whose hearts need special protection against arrhythmias and sudden death.

The special protection program Dr. Lown and his research group have evolved includes medication and psychological counseling. Since there is no good way to determine ahead of time which antiarrhythmic drug will work in a particular patient, the first stage of the protection program begins with acute drug testing—an approach, Dr. Lown said, that permits him to narrow the number of available drugs to one in hours instead of waiting days or even weeks. Antiarrhythmic drugs in general act to depress stimulation of the heart by the brain. Dr. Lown has sixteen such drugs in his arsenal—half of them already in general use, the others still experimental.

Stage two is counseling, and because many of Dr. Lown's patients have suffered the harrowing experience of ventricular fibrillation, the first problem to be faced is the psychological trauma that patients invariably have when they realize what has happened to them—and what might happen to them again. Dr. Lown characterizes the psychological effect of having lived through a "sudden death" episode as akin to having a Damoclean sword swaying ominously above one's head. It can be an endless nightmare that some patients suffer through in complete solitude because they do not share it with anybody. Instead, they may deny that it bothers them. But the problem need not be verbalized to exist. Being tired all day or having trouble sleeping or being irritable and not being interested in certain things anymore are all aspects of the tremendous psychological impact of the fear of sudden death.

Coming to terms with the reality of the situation means bringing the patients' fear to the surface so that it no longer is, in Dr. Lown's words, "a submerged anchor pulling them down to the depths of despair." In trying to get his patients to talk about their fears, Dr. Lown has come across all the typical evasive maneuvers. "They say: 'Do we have to talk about it?' Or, 'It's not bothering me.' But their knuckles grow white and their pulse rate goes up —all signs that they are worried and anxious about what has happened to them."

Airing the fears is the best possible thing for the patient to do, Dr. Lown believes, and he and his staff spend a great deal of time trying to get their arrhythmia patients to do just that. They also encourage their patients to get into an exercise program to dissipate anxiety and they teach them a relaxation technique based on breathing exercises.

With these psychological techniques and with appropriate antiarrhythmic drugs, about 80 percent of Dr. Lown's patients who have been revived from sudden death have been protected from a recurrence—some over a period of five years, a mean time for all of twenty-two months. This contrasts with a 35 percent mortality in two years for a comparable group of patients in Seattle who had received antiarrhythmic medication but not psychological counseling.

The relaxation technique used as the cornerstone in the Harvard program is based on the progressive relaxation method developed in the 1930s by the physiologist Edmund Jacobsen. The central idea is to maintain a fixed focus, to concentrate on relaxation rather than think. Regis A. DeSilva, M.D., who is the director of Dr. Lown's cardiovascular laboratory and the person responsible for modifying the Jacobsen method for use by arrhythmia patients, admits that professionals and hard-nosed business types ("sophisticated people you wouldn't think would go for something like this") begin to see the relevance of their emotional lives to their illness, and they realize something has to be done. His relaxation-technique instructions, which he advises patients to follow twice a day, are:

1. Sit quietly in a comfortable position.
2. Take a deep breath and hold it.
3. Close your eyes.
4. Let out your breath all the way and start breathing quietly.
5. Relax all your muscles, beginning at your face and progressing down to your toes. Keep them relaxed.
6. Breathe through your nose. Become aware of your breathing. As you breathe out, say the word "breathe" silently to yourself. For example, breathe in . . . out . . . "breathe"; in . . . out . . . "breathe," etc.
7. Continue for twenty minutes. You may open your eyes to

check the time, but do not use the alarm. When you finish, sit quietly for several minutes at first with closed eyes and later with your eyes open.

8. Do not worry about whether you are successful in achieving relaxation. Maintain a passive attitude and permit relaxation to occur at its own pace. When distracting thoughts occur, ignore them and continue repeating "breathe."

9. Do not relax immediately after a meal. Wait about two hours before relaxing.

10. Do not lie down while relaxing or you may fall asleep.

This type of relaxation is a way of shutting off excess input to the heart—input that constantly bombards it from the sympathetic nervous system when a person is fully alert and attuned to the distractions, anxieties, noise and demands that ordinarily jangle the nerves and impinge on the heart. The success of this technique, combined with antiarrhythmic drugs has been—no pun intended—heartening, and it has led researchers to look to the brain to protect the heart.

Dr. Lown's group has been investigating ways to increase the brain's concentration of serotonin, a natural substance that acts to reduce nerve traffic to the heart, in an effort to contain the hypothetical trigger of arrhythmias that lurks somewhere within the brain's convoluted borders. Dr. Lown himself envisions a day in the future "when a patient's brain and hormonal function will be monitored continuously by computers as he talks with a counselor ferreting out the sources of neural impulses which accelerate the heartbeat or change the electrophysiological properties of the heart." The computer would then provide a map of the "emotional hotspots" and therapy could concentrate on moderating their effect on the heart.

Until that day—and even presumably beyond it—medical researchers, such as Dr. Lown, will continue as they have in the past decades to pursue methods for controlling and preventing unusual and sometimes life-threatening disturbances in the heart's rhythm, an effort that has already proven remarkably successful.

14

ANGINA

Michael Farley began his personal battle against heart disease in 1971 when he turned forty. He should have started sooner.

His commitment to reduce the risk factors for heart disease brought him to his family doctor for a checkup and his first serum cholesterol test. He did not get comforting news as a birthday present. His cholesterol level was elevated to above 300; he was a good twenty pounds overweight, according to the charts; his blood pressure was way too high. And his heredity was working against him: his father had died instantly of a massive heart attack at the age of forty-nine.

You might say the cards were stacked against Michael Farley, though he did not look at it that way. As an electronics engineer working on the design of new computers, he was in the midst of a booming industry in Massachusetts. His two boys were happy. His was a warm and loving family. He did his best to lower his cholesterol level by maintaining a low-fat diet, but he figures that it did more to help his wife stay trim than it helped him because he had a hard time sticking to it. His red hair might be thinning a bit, but he felt great, and he never had a twinge of chest pain.

Eight years passed. His sons turned into teen-agers. Perhaps his hair got a little thinner on top and a little grayer. If he thought about heart disease, it was only because he was approaching the age at which his father had died. He still felt fine. There were no outward signs that he was otherwise. None, that is, until one weekend a couple of years ago when he had been working in the yard. He remembers how tired he felt, struggling to remove a dead branch from a tree. It could have been the effects of creeping age, or maybe he was letting himself get a little too out of shape. A few minutes' rest would take care of it. He headed inside, to the living room and to the distraction of reading the newspaper.

You can almost picture him sitting there with the newspaper: Michael Farley, age forty-eight, six feet even, 190 pounds, light complexion, blue eyes. His voice was strident as the newspaper dropped from his hands, and the long, open *a*'s typical of the Boston accent must have been particularly drawn out as he called to his wife, Mary, in an adjacent room. He felt a tightening in his chest, and he thought that some of the sandwich he was eating had come back up and caught in his throat. He sipped at the glass of water Mary had drawn in the kitchen. Ten, fifteen minutes later, it was as if nothing had happened. His first encounter with angina might just as well have been indigestion for all the significance Michael Farley gave it.

His second encounter, only a few hours later, did not go quite as casually. The time was around midnight, and Michael was in bed, nearly asleep. This time there was no mistaking what was happening. The pain spread down the length of his left arm. He could barely sit up. Mary got their doctor on the phone. His message was terse: Call the Concord rescue squad.

Police and emergency medical technicians arrived within minutes. Michael Farley got Concord's quickest service, but his pains had stopped before his would-be rescuers had a chance to do anything. For safety's sake, the decision was made to take him to the hospital.

If he thought, as many people with chest pain do, that "Oh my God, I've got angina, the world's coming to an end," he never let on, for in truth, Mike did not know what had happened to him beyond the fact that he could have had a heart attack. He was to learn later, in the hospital, that what he had was a warning. For that is what angina is: a warning that the heart muscle is not getting enough blood. It tells you to stop whatever you are doing and take precautions.

The first misconception about angina is that it is a disease. It is not. Angina is a symptom; in other words, a sensation caused by some underlying disorder. In the case of angina, the underlying disorder is almost always coronary artery disease, although anemia or a constriction in the aorta due to emotional distress also can cause it. According to Peter F. Cohn, M.D., director of the clinical cardiology service at Boston's Peter Bent Brigham Hospital, the sensation itself may not be the "classical" pain directly under the breastbone that everyone's heard about. The pain can start as an ache in the arms or the jaw, or it can mimic indigestion. By and large, though, anginal pains do not occur until the blood flow within a coronary artery has been reduced by at least 60 percent, and a portion of the heart muscle is taxed to the point that it uses up all the available oxygen supplied to it by the narrowed vessel. This was the situation Mike Farley's doctors suspected had brought him to the hospital, and the situation that, very possibly, may have saved his life.

Had his anginal warning system been, in a sense, defective, as it is in certain people who, for some still unknown reason, do not get anginal pains when they should, Mike might have been home rather than in the hospital when he had an "even more serious episode," as his doctor euphemistically characterized the third attack. Mike recalls it more explicitly: "It was like someone sticking a knife in my chest and twisting the blade."

Thousands of people with angina never have a heart attack. Thousands of others with angina eventually do. There is no way of telling beforehand who will fall into which group. Mike Farley's third anginal attack turned into a heart attack. The lack of blood supply could have been temporary, as it had been the day before. No one knows why it was not. Nor does anyone know why the shutoff lasted so long the third time. But it did, and Mike Farley's heart has a small patch of dead muscle as a result.

Of her husband's seventeen-day hospitalization, Mary Farley remembers most clearly seeing him the first day in the intensive care unit: "Even with the tubes and wires in him, he could still smile and he had some joking things to say to the kids. I, myself, was frantic." Later on she experienced fear about taking him home, fear about what she could do if something more happened. He did not stay awake long at night those first few weeks after leaving the hospital. At night, in bed, she found herself listening to his breathing. "He'd lay on his back and snore quite a bit, then sometimes he seemed to hold his breath awhile and I would wonder if he might stop breathing."

Mary Farley regrets that she was not able to share her feelings with others in the same situation during those weeks, but a year afterward she joined a discussion group with a social worker and other spouses of heart patients. "It would have helped a great deal if I had known about such a group and participated even for a short time when I really needed it." As it was, she had to rely on her own hopes for the best, for her husband's heart problems were far from over. Even while he was in the hospital recovering, he had several anginal attacks. There was still heart muscle that was being inadequately supplied with oxygen. The unasked question both Mike and his wife now faced was: Would there be another heart attack?

There were no comforting promises, no assuring answers; there never are. Yet Mike was not left to fend entirely for himself. Angina can be controlled by slowing one's pace of life and by taking medication, and these would be the steps Mike would have to take to ward off a second attack. Even so, there still would be no promises.

The mainstay of angina medication is nitroglycerin, the chemical compound that is known for its explosive properties but that is tame in its medical application. It comes in various forms. One is a tablet, and a single dose usually brings relief in two or three minutes after it is dissolved under the tongue. Nitroglycerin and other members of the nitrate family, which include some long-acting tablets and pads or patches that are worn on the skin and release their medication at a controlled rate for 24 hours, relieve angina by dilating blood vessels and by redistributing the blood supply to the heart muscle so that the regions that need it most get it. When the network of blood vessels throughout the body is suddenly expanded by nitroglycerin, the blood pressure falls and the heart does not have to pump so much blood. The result of these two effects is that the workload of the heart is reduced, and with it, the heart's need for oxygen falls off. Recent research on a third mechanism by which nitroglycerin relieves angina suggests that the drug causes shunting of the blood itself within the heart and that it also relaxes spasms within the wall of a coronary artery.

Beta-blockers, such as propranolol, which depress nervous stimulation of the heart and lower the pulse rate, have been prescribed along with the traditional nitroglycerin. But nitroglycerin is still the only drug that can halt angina in its tracks. In fact, nitroglycerin can be used ahead of time to prevent an angina attack. Patients taking this medication are frequently advised to take it before engaging in any activity (sex, for instance) that they are afraid might trigger the pains.

Some patients decide on their own to wait once their anginal symptoms begin, trying, as Dr. Cohn says, to tough it out. His advice: Don't try it. "It simply does not make sense to suffer for ten to fifteen minutes when the pain will go away in three with nitroglycerin—nor is it wise in a practical medical sense. A person with angina ten times a day is much more likely to get a heart attack than someone having one anginal episode daily. If nitroglycerin prevents those episodes, it is doing something useful."

For Michael Farley, life with angina was neither too precarious nor too different from what it had been. He was told not to climb stairs more than once a day for the first two months out of the hospital, but gradually his cardiologist encouraged more exercise, including an evening walk that eventually extended to two miles.

It was on one of those daily walks several months after he left the hospital that Mike had his first brush with new trouble. "I was walking up a hill near my house and started to puff a bit. The angina came upon me then. As soon as I stopped and rested, it went away, but I took the nitroglycerin tablet anyway." In the two years since that time, he has had only half a dozen anginal episodes, a sign that his condition is under control. He gets winded on long walks and when working in the yard. He does not have the pep that he used to, but, according to his wife, he still is game for almost anything. "He cuts wood and mows the lawn and all that. He's not one who's given up. Each time I see him exerting himself I still get apprehensive. But I know I mustn't try to make a baby out of him. I wouldn't want him to sit around doing nothing."

Michael Farley's efforts in his battle against angina have been largely successful. Tests taken during periodic hospital checkups showed that some of his coronary arteries had narrowings, but they were not so extreme or so placed that they constituted a significant threat to his life. His exercise tolerance also had increased steadily. Had he not done as well and had x-rays of his coronary arteries showed them to be worsening, he might have been advised to have coronary bypass surgery. In this operation, a section of vein, usually removed from the leg (which gets along fine without it), is used to carry blood from the aorta, past the coronary narrowing and back into the coronary, from where it can flow unimpeded into the heart muscle. The extra loop of blood vessel, with one end sutured into the aorta and the other end delicately sutured to the coronary artery, becomes in effect a new coronary artery, and the arteriosclerotic, narrowed section is tied off.

Three months after leaving the hospital, Michael Farley was back at work, exuding his old confidence. "I can handle it perfectly well. It's not stressful, it's interesting, and I don't bring it home with me."

A different perspective comes from Mary Farley:

"He wasn't depressed during his recovery at home, but now his job situation seems to disturb him. There's a lot of change going on in the electronics industry; it's not terribly shaky but I think he wonders where he stands. He knows he can't just go out and get another job—because of his heart attack, and the fact that he's forty-nine years old. During the time he had his heart attack he was overlooked for a position he thinks he could have handled. Maybe the longer he goes with stable health, the better his vocational chances will be."

Perhaps the greatest handicap that Michael Farley and others like him face is the crippling attitude of employers that angina or heart disease disqualifies one for a job. The attitude persists even in a nation that has been led by two Presidents—Dwight D. Eisenhower and Lyndon B. Johnson—who vigorously managed the most demanding job after sustaining heart attacks. Perhaps what heart patients need most is not a better drug, but increased public understanding of how productive someone like Michael Farley can be.

Approximately two million Americans suffer from angina. In some, the symptom of chest pain and the disorder it represents run a fast course, as happened with Michael Farley. Others suffer much longer—years or decades with angina—and they have to confront a number of difficult choices that begin with getting the underlying disorder correctly diagnosed and end with a decision either to undergo bypass surgery or to take medication.

The severity of the angina itself can change, the timing of the pains can change—they can last longer and come more frequently —or the pains can begin to strike during rest, not just during exertion. All of these factors can influence treatment and the decisions that you and your physician will make.

The goal of all treatment for angina, whether it is medical or surgical, is to have the heart's need for oxygen balanced by the supply it receives. This can be accomplished by decreasing the heart's demand for oxygen, and, where appropriate, by relieving spasms that can occur in the coronary arteries.

The coronary arteries normally respond to demands of the heart muscle by dilating or constricting. The only way of bringing more oxygen to the heart muscle under natural circumstances is by widening the coronary arteries, something that happens when exercise or stress puts extra demands on the cardiovascular system. When the demands subside, the coronaries contract.

But what if the arteries contracted more severely and under abnormal circumstances, such as during inactivity or sleep? Researchers speculated that such a contraction could impede the flow of blood to the extent that symptoms of angina might occur.

It was not until the 1970s that coronary artery spasm moved out of the realm of speculation, and for this to happen, several events had to take place.

Albert A. Kattus, M.D., was in attendance as surgeons prepared for coronary artery bypass surgery on a woman who was afflicted with dreadfully painful angina that struck mostly at night while she was asleep. Her heart had just been exposed when one of her coronary arteries did something that no one had ever seen happen, at least at this close range. The artery seemed to clamp down, and Dr. Kattus recalls that when he touched it, it felt like a piece of twine, tough instead of soft and pliable. "We realized," he told an American Heart Association audience in late 1979, "that we had the first eyeball look at an episode of coronary artery spasm any mortal had beheld."

The episode Dr. Kattus described had occurred some years earlier at the hospital of the University of California in Los Angeles. At the time, there was little or no evidence for the existence of coronary artery spasm, although it had been mentioned as early as 1910 and again in 1939 as a possible cause of angina and heart attack. The speculation was that if a coronary artery temporarily contracted for some reason, it would effectively hinder the flow of blood to a portion of the heart muscle in the same way that an arteriosclerotic obstruction of the artery does. Charles K. Friedberg, M.D., and Henry Horn, M.D., the two physicians who had proposed the idea of coronary artery spasm in the *Journal of the American Medical Association* in 1939, suggested that spasm had been responsible for initiating heart attacks in some of their patients, but the spasm theory took a back seat as other causes of heart attack—particularly the arteriosclerotic-plaque theory—gained credence in the 1940s and 1950s.

Doctors believed that a combination of plaques and clots was solely responsible for cutting off a portion of the blood supply to the heart, and they were supported in this belief by experimental evidence as well as by post-mortem examinations. Angina occurs, they said, when the heart's demand for oxygen-rich blood increases during physical exertion, emotional upheaval or other stresses, but a blockage in one or more coronary arteries impedes the flow.

This seemed to make perfectly good sense until 1959, when cardiologist Myron Prinzmetal, M.D., of Los Angeles, California, published case histories of some of his patients who suffered angina while they rested or slept and not while they were exerting themselves. This variation, which has come to be called Prinzmetal's angina, could not be accounted for by the conventional arteriosclerotic-plaque theory, and Dr. Prinzmetal resurrected the notion of coronary artery spasm. This time the theory stuck. But it still lacked one important element. If spasms actually do occur, the skeptical view held, then someone ought to see one happen during surgery or during special x-ray studies of the coronary arteries.

That is indeed what happened. In 1973 Philip B. Oliva, M.D., then chief of cardiology at Denver General Hospital, managed to get x-ray proof of a coronary artery in spasm during an attack of Prinzmetal's angina in one of his patients. Additional evidence came from the University of Pisa in Italy, where Attilio Maseri, M.D., who has since moved to the Royal Postgraduate Medical

School at Hammersmith Hospital in London, England, performed special diagnostic tests that implicated spasm in both Prinzmetal's and exertional angina. Dr. Maseri also discovered that coronary artery spasm, which could last for seconds or minutes, could produce severe arrhythmias, and he found strong circumstantial evidence suggesting that spasm can cause a heart attack.

The cause of spasm itself, though, is still unclear. Psychological stress and cigarette smoking are suspects, as is the potent vascular constrictor thromboxane A_2 that is released by blood platelets. Spasm, either alone or in combination with arteriosclerotic coronary artery disease, is now firmly established as a factor in the complex scenario of heart disease, and researchers are investigating ways to combat it. One of the most promising is calcium antagonism. It is known that calcium, which exists normally within cells as well as in the fluid that bathes them, is necessary for muscular contraction. A substance that could block the movement of calcium into cells could, it is believed, thwart coronary artery spasm and cause dilation of the arteries. Two such drugs, the calcium antagonists nifedipine and verapamil, are being used for patients who cannot get relief from their anginal discomfort solely using the traditional nitroglycerin medication. Calcium antagonists, also known as calcium channel blockers, are effective dilators of coronary arteries. Ordinary aspirin, which blocks the clumping of platelets and therefore, theoretically, the release of thromboxane A_2, may also turn out to be an effective medication to inhibit spasm.

Diagnostic tests that can provoke a coronary artery spasm in angina patients have also been developed, but because of the danger they pose, these tests (known as the cold pressor test and ergonovine challenge) are performed only in hospitals where the patient can be rapidly resuscitated in case the spasm triggers an arrhythmia. Such tests not only provide a way to identify angina patients who are susceptible to spasm but also permit researchers to gauge the effectiveness of new drugs that are being developed to treat it.

15

HEART BLOCK AND THE ARTIFICIAL PACEMAKER

On a narrow neck of land jutting out from the shore of Martha's Vineyard sits a two hundred-year-old weather-beaten house surrounded by prim gardens and lush flower beds. When the season is right and the earth is warm enough to be tilled, a stooped white-haired figure can be seen tending the plants and coaxing out the weeds. On closer inspection he turns out to be a ruddy-faced, healthy-looking man, about five foot six, with a bit of a paunch. There is nothing outwardly obvious about him or about the way he tends to his business that would lead a casual observer to suspect that his heart had given out several times in the past.

Originally a florist, later a librarian, Nelson Coon writes, gardens, takes care of his housekeeping chores and occasionally makes the ferry ride to the Massachusetts mainland to give a lecture or attend a flower show. "When I retired at the age of sixty, I determined I was going to work until I was ninety-six, and I think I'll be able to do it," he says with an infectious grin. He does not have all that long to go, for he was born in 1895.

If Nelson Coon makes it, he will be able to thank not only his irrepressible spirit, but also an electrical device that has been tending to his own heart since the late 1960s. On the right wall of his chest, just south of his collarbone, is a roundish bulge the size of a pocket watch where his artificial pacemaker is implanted just beneath the skin. For fifteen years, while he wrote six books, conducted tours of the great gardens of Europe and otherwise led a full and active life, such a unit has kept his heart at a steady 68–70 beats a minute. Occasionally, before he had it installed, his heart rate would drop into the 20s, and even stop entirely for a second or two at a time. Without the pacemaker, Mr. Coon might well be pushing up daisies instead of writing about them.

The need for such a device became apparent one day in downtown Vineyard Haven as Mr. Coon was headed toward the post office. The letter he was about to mail blew away from his grasp, and when he bent down to recover it, he blacked out. He did not regain consciousness for half an hour, and he ended up in Peter Bent Brigham Hospital. Tests pinpointed the damage in the tiny, delicate conductive fibers that carry minute electrical pulses to the ventricles for coordinating the heart's rhythm. According to his physician, Paul J. Axelrod, M.D., a Boston cardiologist and Harvard Medical School professor, Mr. Coon did not suffer a heart attack. His coronary arteries were fine for a man his age, and no portion of his heart had been subjected to a lack of oxygen. Nevertheless, his heart had been affected by a degenerative aging process that progressively damaged the conduction system. In other words, it was simply the ravages of time that had caused some of the conduction fibers to wear out, and fibrous tissue, which is ineffective in transmitting electrical signals, had formed in their place.

Somewhere, either in the fibers that carried the impulses from Mr. Coon's natural pacemaker (the sinoatrial node) or in the fibers that fan out from the relay node in the wall between his two ventricles, a temporary interruption occurred and the signal was delayed in getting through to the main pumping chambers. The result was that his heart temporarily slowed to the point that not enough blood was pumped to his brain to maintain consciousness.

Ordinarily, the heart's main electrical signal races from a node in the upper right atrium along three special conduction pathways to the auxiliary node in the septum, and from there into the ventricles themselves. This dual-node arrangement allows the atria to contract a fraction of a second before the ventricles, and this, in turn, accounts for the smooth flow of blood through the heart's four chambers. When an interruption occurs in the signal at any point along the conduction pathway—as it did in Mr.

Coon's heart—the resulting condition is known as "heart block." Depending on the severity of the transmission delay, some or all of the impulses from the top of the heart are blocked from reaching the lower half, either temporarily or permanently. In some people the control center for the lower part of the heart takes over the timing for the ventricles, but usually at a very slow pace—perhaps 35 beats a minute or less. Hence, Nelson Coon's occasional slow pulse and fainting spell. In others, the lower control center itself fails, and the ventricles stop beating.

To avert such potentially life-threatening conditions, doctors since 1960 have had a nearly perfect solution: the artificial pacemaker, a compact and remarkable device that is designed to transmit impulses directly to the heart either continuously or whenever the heart's natural signal goes awry. Nelson Coon is one of more than 400,000 people around the world (half of them Americans) whose hearts are regulated by one type of pacemaker or another. Of his pacemaker, Mr. Coon says, "I can't feel it unless I reach my hand up and touch it. There it is and that's it and that's the end of it. I haven't felt any better or any worse as a result of it, but it has prevented me from any further lapses of heart action, which I'm told could be fatal. It's a perfect answer to the problem."

Had Nelson Coon's heart block been continuous rather than temporary, he might have noticed a more dramatic change in his life once his pacemaker had been inserted. A continuous heart block can permanently reduce the heart's action from a normal rate of 72 beats a minute to a sluggish 30 beats a minute. (Unlike a well-conditioned athlete or marathon runner, whose *resting* heart rate may be in the 30s or 40s per minute, a person with heart block is unable to increase his heart rate.) With a heart rate that slow, every minor exertion can cause shortness of breath. That is what happened to another of Dr. Axelrod's patients. Harold Beasely was eighty-one years old when his heart rate dropped so precipitously that he was barely able to move about. His circulation had slowed, his legs had become swollen and he was in heart failure by the time Dr. Axelrod saw him. Diagnostic tests revealed the problem to be heart block. A pacemaker was inserted, and Mr. Beasely recalls that immediately "the pulse rate came right up; I felt much better." In the following weeks he found that he could do more. "I'm no jogger or anything—I'm not entering the Boston Marathon—but I get around fine. I go to the store, get my meals, wash the dishes, walk a little every day."

He also takes his pulse for a full minute a day to check on the functioning of his pacemaker, a recommendation made by pacemaker manufacturers and by many but not all cardiologists. Mr. Beasely's pacemaker is set at a steady 70 beats a minute night and day. If it drops down to 68—a sign that the battery is running down—the pacemaker handbook recommends that he call his doctor to make arrangements for the insertion of a fresh battery pack or a new pacemaker. If it drops to 66, the booklet tells him, he should see his physician immediately.

Thousands of other pacemaker users get monthly long-distance medical assurance by having their devices checked, in effect, by phone. An article in a publication from Medtronics, a pacemaker manufacturer, tells of a Chicago businessman who was granted permission by his doctors to travel for weeks in Europe only if he allowed them to monitor his heart rate at regular intervals. Seated comfortably in his Paris hotel room, he put on snug metal bracelets connected by wires to a device he had brought with him—a special unit housed in an attaché case, used to send a tracing of his heart's activity by telephone. He called his doctor's office back home in Chicago and activated the transmitter by placing the telephone receiver in a special cradle in the case. A unit at the other end translated the signals from Paris into an electrocardiograph tracing of peaks and valleys that indicated a perfectly normal beat. Within minutes, the specialist in Chicago had read the evidence and called back to say that everything looked fine.

For some pacemaker users, the 1-inch-thick, 5-oz. device that is implanted in their chest seems like a time-bomb silently ticking away. They are overly conscious of the bulge beneath their collarbone, and they are constantly worried about the possibility that a machine that their lives are dependent on may malfunction. Reassurance from other pacemaker users helps to a degree, but Dr. Axelrod discourages his patients from taking their pulse rate or from following any regular procedure that would remind them of their pacemakers. "I want them to think of themselves as well people, not heart patients," he says.

The vast majority of pacemaker users will not die even if their pacemakers stop functioning entirely (which is highly unlikely).

Some may have no ill effects, while some others may have a return of symptoms. Dr. Axelrod estimates that only one of his patients out of ten would be in serious danger if the pacemaker were turned off abruptly. Many patients in whom this has happened have lived through it.

There are two types of pacemaker failure. The first is abrupt termination caused if a wire breaks or the power supply suddenly malfunctions. This cannot be predicted by pulse taking or by telephone monitoring. The second type is gradual weakening of the power cell, which can be detected and forecast by the doctor when he examines the patient at three-month intervals. "So why should the patient be burdened," Dr. Axelrod asks, "with the concern about catastrophic malfunction if malfunction would lead to mild or no symptoms and is usually predictable anyway?"

It is a rhetorical question, and in Dr. Axelrod's view patients clearly need not bother monitoring their pacemakers by taking their pulse. However, there is another school of thought on this issue. Although some cardiologists agree with Dr. Axelrod, other cardiologists believe that daily monitoring of the pulse is comforting to a patient who has been concerned about heart rate all along. They, as well as the American Heart Association, recommend daily pulse taking.

Harold Beasely followed that recommendation, and he was certainly no worse off for it. Nelson Coon, on the other hand, turned out to be one of Dr. Axelrod's ideal patients, for he is adamant about *not* taking his pulse. "Oh, heavenly days, I wouldn't consider it under any circumstances. I don't take any precautions, none at all. I don't do anything at all except go about my work."

Neither Mr. Coon nor Mr. Beasely required a pacemaker because of damage suffered during a heart attack. In this respect they are typical of most pacemaker users. A heart attack, however, can create the need for a pacemaker. The crucial fibers carrying signals from the upper to the lower part of the heart are confined in a very narrow pathway within the wall of tissue separating the right and left sides of the heart. If a portion of that wall becomes injured or swollen, the result may be either temporary or permanent interruption of the conduction system. This happens in 5 percent of all heart attacks. A temporary, external pacemaker, which sends its signal through a wire within a catheter that is inserted into an arm vein and threaded into the heart, can be used to boost the heart rate. If the heart recovers its natural rhythm, the wire is simply removed; if not, a permanent pacemaker is installed.

Another condition that calls for a pacemaker is the "sick sinus syndrome," in which the heart's natural pacemaker transmits impulses too slowly. Even the point at which the impulse for the beat originates tends to wander within the atrium of the heart. The resulting conduction disturbance causes a decrease in the heart rate, which may be experienced as angina, and a concomitant decrease in the volume of blood that is pumped from the heart. By diminishing the supply of oxygen to the brain, sick sinus syndrome produces symptoms that may be falsely attributed to senility or minor strokes, including fainting spells, slight personality changes, irritability, memory loss and insomnia in the early stages and, later, slurred speech, slight paralysis and faulty judgment.

The installation of a permanent, internal pacemaker is not a major operation. It takes no more than an hour and a half and is generally performed under local anesthesia, commonly in a special-procedures room with x-ray equipment that permits the surgeon to observe his progress as he guides the wire leading from the pacemaker through a vein and into the heart. Most pacemakers are inserted under the skin in the upper right-hand corner of the chest, but occasionally they are placed in the upper left portion of the abdominal cavity, with the wire then attached to the outer surface of the heart muscle. The reason for the lower placement in the abdomen instead of on the surface of the chest may be physical, as in the case of children whose small veins make the upper placement impractical, or it may be cosmetic, as in the case of a woman who does not want to wear a bathing suit or an evening gown with a bump on her chest.

As has been mentioned, the power source for pacemakers does not last forever (Mr. Coon has had his replaced four times in the last fifteen years). When the battery eventually runs down, the entire device, short of the wires that attach it to the heart, must be replaced in a half-hour procedure that necessitates a day or less in the hospital. Pacemakers have undergone steady improvement since the devices first came into general use in 1960. Technological advances in the power source and in the materials used to enclose the pacemaker itself have greatly increased their usefulness, and electronics specialists have designed a variety of types to fit particular needs. The "on-demand" pacemaker, which shuts off whenever the heart beats properly on its own, is an improvement over the previous, automatic pacemaker, which ignored any spontaneous beats of the heart. The "on-demand" pacemaker is, however, sensitive to some types of electrical signals emanating from such equipment as metal detectors, which are used for security checks at airports and other public installations. The electricity generated by the detector might be interpreted by the pacemaker as a natural impulse from the heart itself, temporarily causing the pacemaker to shut off. Pacemaker users are therefore advised to request a manual search instead. Diathermy equipment that is used in hospitals, microwave-cooking apparatus, and such things as electric razors or electric tools should all be used with caution or not at all.

Another version of the "on-demand" pacemaker senses the natural beat of the heart's upper chambers, which frequently beat normally even though electrical flow to the lower heart is blocked, and relays this information to the ventricles, which then adopt the upper chambers' pace. If a person with this type of pacemaker starts walking after a period of rest, his heart's upper chambers will naturally accelerate to, let's say, 80 beats per minute, and his ventricular rate will simultaneously increase to that level, an effect that does not happen with the older "on-demand" pacemakers. The obvious benefit is that the heart is able to respond to changing physical demands in a more natural, physiological way.

The newest pacemakers can also be reset to run faster or slower by electrical signals from outside the body, and they send out warning signals when their batteries are about to fail. Researchers are, in fact, developing pacemakers that incorporate the latest in microcomponent technology, which has already revolutionized the electronics industry. They have begun testing pacemakers that are designed around the miniature components of a computer—a central processing unit, memory, and reprogrammable instructions—that will give future pacemakers tremendous flexibility and a range of functions much broader than just generating an impulse when the heart's own signal fails.

Dr. Axelrod expects that it will not be long before pacemakers are able to store the medical history of a patient and to transmit it on a signal for instant print-out. Future pacemakers might very well have the capacity to monitor the electrical activity of the heart and store samples of normal and abnormal rhythms, and it is conceivable that sensors could be built in so as to monitor blood pressure and chemicals in the blood that are vital to the electrical conduction system of the heart. Pacemakers may be employed to correct too rapid heartbeats and other arrhythmias, either automatically or on command from the pacemaker user. An implanted defibrillator has already been developed to protect those at risk from sudden death. Pacemaker scientists are currently at work developing devices to manage both these problems, but there are still unanswered questions about the physiology of the heart that have to be explored before such devices are given widespread clinical application.

In the meantime, for hundreds of thousands of people, pacemakers are the perfect treatment. After all, what other form of treatment shuts itself off when it is not needed and turns itself on when it is?

16

CONGESTIVE HEART FAILURE

In the late 1700s, around the time of the American Revolution, a gentleman who may have been a professor—the records are not clear on this point—living at one of the colleges that had made Oxford, England, renowned throughout the educated world, became ill with a condition that was known as dropsy. This is a swelling of the tissues, frequently starting in the legs and gradually progressing to the lungs as the heart's pumping action weakens and fails to keep the blood moving adequately. Through the grapevine, this gentleman heard of a cure for his condition offered by an aged midwife skilled in herbal brews. He journeyed to her home, where he was given a packet of the homemade remedy and instructions on how to prepare it, which were not unlike those for steeping ordinary tea. Once he had begun drinking the midwife's mixture, his condition dramatically improved, his swellings diminished and his heart pumped with renewed vigor.

Word of his recovery and of the potion's remarkable curative properties reached a doctor in Birmingham who would figure prominently in this story, in 1775. William Withering, the physician in question, began a careful analysis of the mixture's ingredients, and after having tested the active ones on several of his private patients who happened to be suffering from dropsy, concluded that of the twenty or more different herbs in the brew, only one was active against the waterlogging of dropsy. This came from the plant called foxglove, or, as it had been described botanically two hundred years earlier, *Digitalis purpurea*, for its flower, which is purple and resembles, by a stretch of the imagination, a finger. "It has a power over the motion of the heart to a degree yet unobserved in any other medicine," Dr. Withering wrote in his *Account of the Foxglove*, published in London in 1785, "and this power may be converted to salutory ends." His foresight was not fully recognized until the 1920s, when digitalis became the keystone in the treatment of the modern-day equivalent of dropsy, now known as congestive heart failure, or, simply, heart failure.

It is, perhaps, one of the more unfortunate terms in the lexicon of medical diagnosis because of its frightening implications: *heart failure.* The term itself seems to suggest extinction. So thought Margaret Kelly when she learned that her heart was failing. "I almost passed out; I figured my time had come," she said, looking back on the day that diagnosis was made. That was five years ago, but her ordeal had actually begun three years earlier when she started noticing symptoms that her doctor later told her were indicative of the first stage of congestive heart failure. Her feet and ankles, she recalled, would be swollen at the end of the day—so much so that if she took off her shoes she could not put them on again. Yet at the time she did not take the condition seriously, for the swelling disappeared when she slept and she had no idea that her heart was involved.

She had had similar episodes of swollen feet in the past, after she had been standing a great deal or after she had been sitting in a plane for several hours on her annual Christmas flight to visit her daughter, and like most women, she had experienced edema years earlier when she was pregnant and during the days immediately preceding her menstrual period, which she knew was no cause for alarm. However, had she mentioned the sudden recurrence of these symptoms to her doctor, she might have been spared the second stage of heart failure, which occurred three years later when the fluid that had been accumulating in her body finally appeared in her lungs.

She knew something was drastically wrong when she became breathless climbing the stairs to her apartment—something that had never occurred before—and when she found breathing difficult in bed without several extra pillows propping up her head. Prompted by these symptoms, she finally sought medical help. As she was to learn from her doctor, in the ensuing days during which she had chest x-rays and an electrocardiogram, all her symptoms over the past three years were linked to her heart, and its condition had been growing worse in recent months. However, with every increment in the severity of her problem in the months before she saw her doctor, she had found a way to combat the symptoms of her slowly failing heart. Resting and raising her legs after a long day decreased the swelling, so she belittled the problem. If it went away, she thought to herself, then how serious could it be? Sleeping on a stack of pillows tilted her lungs, concentrating the fluid that had accumulated in them into a smaller area so that she was no longer drowning in it, no longer experiencing a feeling of suffocation. But no matter how hard she had tried to put this out of her mind, it began troubling her. Why, she wondered, was she having a hard time breathing? It was something she could not ignore.

Thwarting the symptoms of congestive heart failure, though, does nothing to thwart a failing heart. Had Margaret Kelly waited to seek medical attention weeks or even days later than she did, her condition might have deteriorated to the more ominous stages of congestive heart failure in which it is impossible to sleep without becoming desperately short of breath, to the point of rushing to the window and flinging it open to get some air. In its final stage, a frothy blood-tinged fluid chokes off nearly all the air to the lungs, which, barring prompt treatment with drugs and oxygen, is fatal.

Congestive heart failure, which means simply that the heart is unable to pump enough blood for the body to function well, is usually the result of a diseased heart—most often, as in Mrs. Kelly's case, caused by coronary artery disease. But other heart conditions, such as an actual heart attack or leaky or narrowed heart valves, due to rheumatic and congenital heart disease, can also lead to failure. About 10 percent of heart attack victims who are discharged from the hospital after recuperating have to take medication for congestive heart failure due to the residual damage to the ventricles which restricts fully effective pumping. Other conditions, however, require more drastic therapy. If the damage causing the heart failure is a cardiac aneurysm (a bulge due to thinning of the wall of the left ventricle), surgical repair may be necessary to remove the weakened section of muscle and eliminate the source of the problem. Surgery is also the answer for heart failure that is caused by damaged heart valves.

In mitral stenosis, for instance, the leaflets of the mitral valves are fused more or less together (often as the result of rheumatic fever which occurred during the patient's childhood), obstructing the flow of blood between the left atrium and left ventricle and causing a characteristic heart murmur, as the snapping sound of the damaged mitral valve trying to open reverberates in a low-pitched, rumbling sound best heard at the bottom of the heart. Pressure readings within the left ventricle, measured with a special catheter that is threaded backward through an artery into the left ventricle and left atrium, help not only to confirm the diagnosis but also to assess the extent of the heart's impairment. If the valve is still fairly flexible, the surgeon may be able to repair it by separating the leaflets, but if they are heavily calcified or too misshapen, he will have to replace them with an artificial valve.

Among still other causes of heart failure are a category of puzzling disorders known as cardiomyopathies (literally, heart muscle diseases) that are not related to arteriosclerosis. These include some caused by toxins like alcohol, some produced by viruses, and some caused by deposits of either iron or an abnormal body substance called amyloid in the heart tissue itself. No one knows the fundamental reason why millions of cardiac muscle cells begin weakening from these various heart ailments—researchers are searching for answers—but when they do, the heart's pumping action weakens and circulation slows, setting off an internal domino effect that gradually topples every organ in the body if it is not halted in time.

With inadequate circulation, the kidneys fail to excrete enough water, salt and waste substances. Consequently, the blood volume increases, producing more work for the already overburdened heart, which may enlarge and beat faster in a desperate attempt to meet the body's demand for oxygen-rich blood. Veins become swollen, and the balance of hydrostatic pressures between the fluids inside and outside these vessels shifts, causing fluid that normally stays in the bloodstream to leak into the surrounding tissue. This fluid first accumulates in the legs, and later on in the lungs, where it causes shortness of breath.

Margaret Kelly's heart failure had progressed through these stages, as was evident to her doctor after a brief physical examination, but the full extent of the damage became clear only after chest x-rays, an echocardiogram and an ECG. The x-rays showed that her heart's left and right ventricles were enlarged and her electrocardiogram showed signs of heart muscle damage caused by disease of her coronary arteries.

The damage was irreparable. Her heart would never again function at the high level it once did, but it could continue to function at a reduced level for many years with proper treatment, and that is precisely what her doctor set out to accomplish. The treatment of a failing heart is directed toward two objectives: first, to help the heart pump more efficiently, and second, to decrease its workload by reducing the amount of blood it has to pump and the resistance against which the heart pumps.

Digitalis, the drug derived from the foxglove plant, and newer drugs like it increase the vigor of contraction of the heart's muscle fibers, causing the ventricles to pump more powerfully—in effect, more efficiently. While the drug has direct effect on increasing the blood flow to the kidneys, another class of drugs, the diuretics, is used to stimulate the kidneys to excrete excess salt and water that accumulate in heart failure. Both drugs work hand in hand to reduce the heart's burden.

Like thousands of heart-failure patients before her, Mrs. Kelly was advised to restrict her salt intake. Salt tends to increase edema because the body has to dilute the salt with fluid, chiefly water, which it draws out of the circulatory system into the surrounding tissue. This meant avoiding not only table salt, but also the sodium chloride in soda crackers and the sodium nitrite in bacon, lunchmeat and sausages. She was advised to replace commercially processed foods, which tend to be salty, with fresh vegetables; and she learned to use herbs and spices to perk up the flavor of her food. The medication she was taking, she recalled, worked like magic, and she was able to be more active without getting tired, to sleep soundly without fear of suffocation. Whenever she felt unduly tired, she stopped and sat down and rested, as she was advised to do. As she improved, she took daily walks.

Although exercise does not reverse congestive heart failure, it can improve the heart's efficiency just as exercise does for a heart that is not in failure. However, there are types of heart failure in which exercise can be dangerous, even lethal. If the heart failure is caused by narrowing of the heart's aortic valve (a condition known as aortic stenosis), exercise can lead to fainting or sudden death. The word of caution here is to follow the advice of your doctor, who is the best judge of whether or not you should exercise.

One of the significant advances in preventing congestive heart failure has been, in a roundabout way, medication that is used to treat high blood pressure. In the years before doctors could control high blood pressure with drugs, this condition would often progressively weaken the heart to the point of failure. Now that is not so often the case. Diuretics and vasodilators (which expand arteries all over the body) can lower the blood pressure and ward off the strain it puts on the heart. And even when long-term heart failure is due to causes other than high blood pressure, vasodilators have become part of the standard treatment, because advanced failure by itself can lead to excessive arterial constriction.

"The real solution to heart failure," concludes Edgar Haber, M.D., chief of cardiology at Massachusetts General Hospital, "will not be in the realm of better drugs or other treatments for this condition. We must first find out the exact mechanism which causes the heart-muscle cell to fail. What does failure really mean? Why are some hearts able to withstand prolonged high blood pressure without failing? Heart failure is the reaction of the heart to something else, not really a disease in itself. We must solve it ultimately by solving its primary causes—just as it's far better to avoid an automobile accident than it is to repair the injured body that results from the accident."

17

THE BYPASS

It was eight o'clock on a hot July morning in Kansas City, Missouri. Clay Farnes, forty-four, was lying on an operating table in St. Luke's Hospital awaiting surgery for severely obstructed coronary arteries. Just before losing consciousness, he overcame the inebriated silliness induced by the pre-operation injection long enough to utter aloud a prayer for survival. It seemed appropriate under the circumstances. Clay's younger brother, a stockbroker suffering from chest pains, had been advised by his physician to undergo just such an operation and refused. "They'll kill you in there," he had told his brother, voicing the natural fear of any tampering with the heart, the very symbol of life.

Clay Farnes knew that his heart would have to be stopped—purposefully stilled—during the crucial stage of the operation, and in the days preceding the surgery, whenever the image of his own heart quivering and then lying motionless creeped into his consciousness, he felt a deathly chill in his bones. Richard S. Blacher, M.D., and Richard J. Cleveland, M.D., a psychiatrist and a surgeon, respectively, at Tufts New England Medical Center in Boston, wrote in late 1979 in the *Journal of the American Medical Association* that patients believe they will be dead while the heart is stopped and then brought back to life when it is restarted. The two doctors recognized that this is not an easy misunderstanding to deal with, and while most patients try not to think of it, not all succeed.

Such death fears began surfacing in the 1950s when the development of the heart-lung machine made it possible for surgeons to stop the heart safely and operate on its internal structures—something they had longed to do ever since they realized that most cardiac problems lay beyond their grasp inside the heart itself and not in the nerves and great vessels that surround the heart, which they had been able to operate on prior to an effective heart-lung machine. In fact, operations designed to bring help to an oxygen-starved heart had been attempted as early as the 1920s, but it was not until the mid-1960s, when surgeons devised a way to remove a section of a person's own leg vein and graft it onto a coronary artery, that a successful method was found to reroute blood around an obstruction in the coronary circulation.

Advances in cardiac angiography (an x-ray technique that provides detailed pictures of the internal defects and blockages) allowed surgeons to plan well in advance of the actual operation what they were going to do and how they were going to do it; and the unknowns that had made contemplation of cardiac surgery so difficult and had made the operations themselves so fraught with risks gave way to new optimism and, more important, greater success rates.

Clay Farnes may have had personal misgivings and fleeting fears to contend with, but the operation he was about to undergo, technically known as aortocoronary bypass graft surgery, had successfully weathered much of the criticism against it and by the time of his surgery in 1973 had become a widely accepted procedure for certain heart conditions. It is now the most frequent type of adult heart surgery—as many as four hundred are done on a typical day in United States hospitals—despite the fact that it is one of the most expensive operations. Farnes, who had experienced his first heart attack at the age of thirty-nine, believes it may have saved his life. Five months after Clay's brother warned him about the operation, the brother himself, like his father before him, was dead of a heart attack.

A necessary preliminary to any bypass operation is cine-angiography: x-ray movies of the heart in which the coronary arteries are outlined by a contrast medium injected from the tip of a thin woven plastic catheter that is inserted into the patient's arm or groin and moved through a large artery to the heart itself. As the tip of the catheter enters the aorta, its rate of insertion is slowed, and with the help of a large television screen that amplifies the x-ray image of the heart, it is guided forward until it reaches the opening of the coronary arteries. The tip is then gently pushed into one of the main coronary trunks, and contrast medium that is held in a syringe attached to the external end of the catheter is injected into the artery. Within a second or two, the vessel and its tortuous branches emerge on the screen, looking for all the world like the branches of a scraggly shrub superimposed on the shadow of the beating heart.

In Clay Farnes's angiogram a gap far down the main trunk of the right coronary artery outlined the blockage that had caused his first heart attack. Below the blockage the rest of the vessel—visible because pressure in the coronary arterial tree causes blood and, in this case, contrast medium to backflow to the point of the obstruction—was clear and open, and collateral vessels of the heart's own natural bypass system seemed to be carrying some blood around the obstruction. As contrast medium filled the other main trunks, a moderate to severe narrowing of the vessel appeared halfway down Farnes's left anterior descending coronary artery, and a third appeared in a small diagonal branch leading off from it, both probably the cause of his recent angina. The vascular channels below the obstructions in both the anterior descending coronary and its branch looked perfect for bypass vessels that could bridge the gap, so to speak, around the obstructions in much the same way that traffic is diverted around congested urban centers.

Finally, contrast medium was injected from the catheter tip into the left ventricle, the heart's hardest-working chamber, and x-rays were taken of its pumping action to locate any impaired movements of the heart wall caused by his previous heart attack. But the scar, only an inch in diameter, appeared to make little or no difference. In the days that followed, the angiograms helped his surgeons plan their bypass strategy, and Clay Farnes was given further tests, including more x-rays and blood typing, in anticipation of surgery. Friends telephoned to cheer him, as well as friends of friends—two men who told him about the success of their own bypass operations—and co-workers at Farnes's office donated blood to replace that which would be lost during surgery.

At six o'clock on the morning of the surgery, Farnes awoke to find a phalanx of people standing by his bed. His mother, his wife

Bypassing blocked arteries

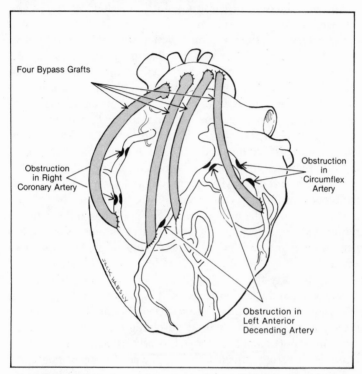

and their son—who would remain in the hospital until the operation was over—and his family physician all offered him emotional support by their presence. When the attendants arrived to take him to surgery, he knew that he had the most important people pulling for him.

On the operating table, anesthetized and with a breathing tube down his throat, Clay Farnes was stripped of his hospital gown, an intravenous line was inserted into an arm vein, and his entire trunk and left leg were scrubbed with yellow antiseptic. A series of three 4-inch incisions was made, starting in his groin and extending down the length of his leg, and an unbroken 15-inch section of a large superficial blood vessel known as the saphenous vein was extracted, bathed in salt water, tested for leaks, and placed in a tray for later use as bypass tubing.

The next incision began at a point just below his throat and followed a straight line down the center of his chest to the diaphragm, exposing the breastbone, which was then opened with a small hand-held stainless-steel oscillating electric saw. As the flanges of a U-shaped metal chest divider forced apart the split chest, Farnes's beating heart, encased in its glistening, fibrous sac, came into view. Tubes from the heart-lung machine were connected to large vessels that carry blood to and from Farnes's heart, in preparation for the moment when his heart would be stopped and his circulation diverted into the plastic coils that weave through the heart-lung machine's curtains of vertical membranes where waste carbon dioxide is removed and oxygen added before the blood's return trip to the body. Once the process begins, the blood—chilled in the machine to 86°F.—cools down the patient's normal 98.6°F. temperature, which, in turn, diminishes the body's need for oxygen and helps the heart-lung machine work more efficiently.

By eight forty-five the heart-lung machine was droning in the background, and Clay Farnes lay still as a statue on the operating table, cold to the touch but rosy-cheeked, his chest forced open a full eight inches, his heart in its glistening sac immobile after an infusion of potassium had stopped its beat. (Potassium blocks the impulses that trigger the heartbeat.) The electroencephalographic tracings of his brain waves, rippling across overhead TV screens, were the only indication that he was alive. The stage was set for the essence of the operation. A thoracic surgeon delicately slit the pericardial sac to expose Farnes's bare heart with its coronary arteries prominently outlined on its surface. The aorta was clamped shut, and a suction line was slipped into the right ventricle to drain the heart of blood. With a small curved needle he attached a portion of the saphenous vein to the left anterior descending coronary artery just below the blockage. Because the small diagonal branch, where the second blockage was lodged, would not match well with the large saphenous vein, the surgeon, using an alternative technique to the conventional bypass, dissected free a small artery that normally nourishes the rib cage and grafted it below the obstruction in the diagonal branch. He did not, however, try to bypass the occlusion in Farnes's right coronary artery because the blockage was at the bottom of the heart where an earlier heart attack had destroyed some muscle and a graft simply would have supplied blood to an area of functionless scar tissue.

Three times an hour, during this tedious, eye-straining suturing, the surgery was halted for five minutes while the aorta was unclamped to allow blood to "give the heart a drink," in the surgeon's words, and supply the cardiac tissue with oxygen. Then to complete the bypass, the free end of the saphenous vein section was sutured around the edges of a small surgical incision made in the aorta. Henceforth, if all went well, the starved heart muscle below the blockage would obtain all the blood it needed via the bypass vessel.

Near noon, the operating team began cleanup and closing. The surgical field was washed with salt water. Clamps were removed to allow blood to flow freely again. The heart was restarted by an electrical shock, and its pericardial sac repaired. The rib cage was allowed to spring back into position, and the breastbone was securely bound together with stainless-steel wires, which would remain permanently embedded in Clay Farnes's chest. The anesthesia was becoming lighter, and Farnes, now nearly awake, felt no pain. He heard someone say, "Let's clean him up," and he remembers something sounding like ethereal music—probably only the background Muzak that pervades even the inner sanctum of some operating rooms. Then the sounds faded, and his next memory was awakening in the recovery room, still heavily sedated, festooned with wires and catheters, annoyed by the breathing tube down his throat that kept him from speaking, but glad to be alive.

For him the next three days in the cardiac intensive care unit flew by in a drugged haze punctuated by the comforting bleeps of the monitor keeping track of his heart and by the ministrations of a stream of nurses, aides and doctors. On the third day he took a supervised walk down the hospital corridor and was moved into a regular room. "I could feel I had been tampered with," he later recalled with characteristic restraint, "but I wasn't really uncomfortable. Except for the soreness, it was a pleasant stay, sort of a vacation." Nine days after the operation he was back home, and in another six weeks he was back at work. Not all bypass patients, as you can guess, are as stoic or as immune to the discomfort and pain that Farnes took in his stride, but in time, the body's remarkable healing powers will take care of all the intrusions of surgery.

What difference has bypass surgery made in the life of Clay Farnes? For months before the operation, he recalled, "I was so tired at the end of the work week that I spent nearly the entire weekend in bed. In the morning I never wanted to get up; I was still exhausted." Almost as soon as he arrived home from the hospital, however, he felt like a new man. "In the morning I wanted to get up, get going, and at night I still had energy to spare." Exercise was not only possible, but fun again. "There was a gentle slope near our house that my wife and I would ascend on our evening walks. Just before my operation I had to stop and rest two or three times just to get to the top. After the bypass surgery I didn't notice the hill. It was as if someone had leveled it."

Those who have undergone bypass surgery since the first reported procedure was performed in 1964 are, in general, enthusiastic about the results. An estimated 165,000 bypass operations were performed in 1981, and the surgery itself is one of the most common, if not the most common, elective surgical procedures performed on adults.

A very few of those who have had bypass surgery have been so improved that they have become marathon runners. Clay Farnes is more typical. Enough of his energy was restored so that he could be reasonably active and enjoy life once more. To him, the operation was a success. "If I had to do it all over again, I would do the same thing," he says.

Yet he knows full well that the operation did not cure him of heart disease (which may or may not be progressing) and that it did not—and could not—undo the damage to his heart caused by his first heart attack. Since his bypass, he has had occasional breathlessness and chest pains, but only after severe exertion. "When we have an emergency around the house," Farnes said, "a leak in the basement or the car stuck in snow, my wife, Mary, cautions me not to overdo, even if it means starting an argument." Mary agreed that she is overprotective at times, but she said that her husband and she have adjusted "pretty well" to their life together since the operation. "We don't go out disco dancing into the late evening, but we still enjoy our daily walk. He gets his eight hours of sleep every night and I prepare only low-cholesterol meals. Our life isn't the same as it once was, but it's just as good."

Clay Farnes worked successfully at his job for a time after the operation, but factors beyond his control made it increasingly stressful, so upon his physician's advice he switched to a low-key occupation in which he sets his own hours—buying, fixing up and selling houses.

What would have happened to Clay Farnes without bypass surgery? No one can say. In the years since the operation he has been almost entirely free of angina, which was incapacitating and unresponsive to medication before the operation. At this writing, he has not had another heart attack, and more to the point, he is alive. According to several major studies, those who receive only medical treatment and not surgery for his condition—blockage of two coronary arteries—die at the rate of 7 percent a year. This jumps to an annual death rate of 12 percent for medically treated disease of the left main coronary artery, which supplies two thirds of the blood to the heart muscle, via the branching circumflex and left anterior descending arteries.

Such figures place in perspective the extremely small mortality rate for the coronary artery bypass procedure when it is performed by highly experienced surgical teams. The cardiac surgeons at St. Luke's, for example, have done more than 4,000 bypass operations in eight years, with a mortality of only 0.8 percent, the same rate as that at the Cleveland Clinic, where the bypass operation was perfected and where surgeons now perform 3,000 bypasses a year. (If a patient's heart has already been damaged by a severe heart attack, his mortality risk may be much higher than average; Clay Farnes was told that his chances of not surviving the operation were about 3 percent.) After evaluating ten years of accumulated evidence, a panel assembled by the National Institutes of Health reached a conclusion late in 1980. Improvements in the bypass procedure within the last few years have made the risk of such surgery virtually negligible compared with the risk of death within the first year for people considered eligible for the bypass.

In the early years of the bypass operation, surgeons could not be sure that it prolonged life—only that it banished angina for most patients and made life more livable. Now, after more than ten years in which hundreds of thousands of bypasses have been done, the evidence is that 90 percent of bypass patients survive for five years. The operation decreases the death rate at least by half —from 10 to 5 percent a year—when it is performed to circumvent a major blockage in the main trunk of the left coronary artery. There is also a 50 percent decline in the death rate after the bypass is performed in people with blockages in the three main coronary arteries. Nonetheless, the story of bypass surgery is not one of total success. Ten percent of bypass grafts close up before the patient leaves the hospital, and only about 70 percent of the grafts are open at the end of three years. Thereafter, the closure rate is 2 percent a year. However, that does not mean that a third of the bypass operations are failures. "It means," according to one surgeon, "that if you have a triple bypass, which is common, you can expect one of them to occlude within three to five years—but you are still better off than before."

Return of angina follows a similar pattern: 75 percent of bypass patients are free of anginal symptoms after one year, but only 60 percent after five years. If the pains return, though, they are often not as severe or as frequent as those experienced before the surgery. And a repeat bypass operation is a possibility.

The role of the bypass, according to the NIH panel, is unclear in patients who are undergoing a heart attack, and the operation is unwarranted in patients who have symptoms but no major blockages in their coronary arteries.

How much are the benefits worth in dollars? The operation is expensive—upwards of $20,000 including hospitalization, medications and laboratory and diagnostic tests—but so is medical treatment for heart disease if a patient has to be hospitalized repeatedly. At Peter Bent Brigham Hospital in Boston, John J. Collins, Jr., M.D., analyzed the hospitalization costs of 102 consecutive bypass surgery patients with chronic, intractable angina. He found that in the two years before surgery, the average patient spent 15.5 days in the hospital; in the two years following surgery, only 3.5 days. The average patient thus saved 5.9 days and $1,770 per year (at 1979 hospital rates averaging a total of $300 per day) following surgery, amortizing the $8,000 hospital portion of the bill in 4.5 years, the physicians' and surgeons' fees in an additional two years or so.

Furthermore, reducing disability, for which the bypass operation has become famous, saves money. Various studies have shown that about 80 percent of bypass patients can resume a normal life following surgery. In a review of 72 heart patients who underwent bypass surgery for obstruction of the left main coronary artery, University of Virginia surgeon Ivan K. Crosby, M.D., found that only 2 were able to work before the operation, but 52 were capable of doing so after surgery, and more than half went back to their previous jobs.

Still, the pros and cons of bypass surgery can be bewildering. Some eminent physicians have publicly questioned the need for most of it, suggesting that many patients would do just as well without surgery by taking today's improved medication. On the other hand, there is a growing conviction among bypass surgeons that the operation, in conditions for which it is indicated, prolongs life and, in the words of Rene C. Favaloro, M.D.—the principal architect of bypass surgery while he was on the staff of the Cleveland Clinic—makes the quality of life "much, much better."

Surgery is frequently recommended when disabling angina cannot be controlled with medication or when the left main coronary artery is blocked (this is the most serious blockage of all, and the one that diminishes circulation to the left ventricle where most heart attack damage occurs) or when more than one of the other coronary arteries are blocked by at least 60 or 70 percent. However, the final decision about whether to undergo bypass surgery can never be based solely on a neat formula. It must take into consideration age—though age itself is not a barrier—other diseases and response to medication, as well as the odds and the alternatives.

For Clay Farnes, the decision boiled down to living free of incapacitating pain or living with crippling angina and the threat of an imminent, possibly fatal heart attack. The development of the successful bypass operation, which has been one of the most illustrious examples of the merger of surgical skills with high technology, offered him—and offers thousands like him—the brighter alternative.

18

VALVULAR DISEASE

Seated behind a desk, he appeared to be of average height. It was only when he stood up, according to his law partner William H. Herndon, that he "loomed above other men," a descriptive phrase about his stature that has come to be justly famous in another context. The bones in his arms and especially those in his legs were abnormally elongated. His fingers seemed to extend beyond a reasonable length. When he brought his outstretched hands together to rest his bearded chin in the angle between his index fingers and his thumbs, as he was apt to do when contemplating the nation's fate, there was a strikingly noticeable aberration between his two hands, as if they belonged to separate people. His left hand towered over his right, particularly in the center where the middle fingers came together.

An astute observer might have noticed that the asymmetry was inconsistent, for casts made of the man's hands in 1860, the year he was first nominated for the presidency, show that his left thumb was a good deal shorter than his right thumb. Those who knew him well kept his difficulties in coordinating and focusing his eyes to themselves. It was an unpopular course to gossip about the Great Emancipator's frailties.

In 1969, more than a century after Abraham Lincoln's assassination, a California physician recognized a stunning similarity in the physical appearance of one of his patients, who happened to be a seven-year-old boy at the time, and that of the Sixteenth President of the United States. The boy, suffering from an inherited connective tissue disorder known as Marfan's syndrome, happened to share a distant ancestor with Lincoln, according to an account in Life Science Library's *Health and Disease*. On the strength of this relationship, and several other medical coincidences between the male members of Lincoln's family, the boy's doctor, Harold Schwartz, M.D., speculated that Lincoln himself suffered from Marfan's syndrome, named for the doctor who first described the ocular, skeletal, and most important, the cardiovascular abnormalities that are associated with the syndrome.

Unbeknownst to those medical practitioners who had remarked upon Lincoln's ungainly skeletal proportions, the President, in all likelihood, was suffering from a weakness of the aorta that is characteristic in Marfan's syndrome, and the attending cardiac problems caused by an incompetent aortic valve well before the time of his assassination. Had that sorrowful event at Ford's Theater not taken place, Lincoln still may not have lived out his second term as President, for doctors at the time could do nothing to repair the aortic valve or, for that matter, any of the heart's other valves.

It was not until the 1960s, after years of experimentation, that surgeons were able to successfully replace damaged valves with artificial substitutes, and while the new valves do not work quite as well as perfectly functioning natural valves, they gave thousands of heart patients a new lease on life. The great majority of patients with valve damage have renewed energy after surgery, and they experience marked improvement in the way they feel.

Of the heart's four valves, the two on the hard-working left side of the heart are most likely to need replacement. The mitral valve, located between the left atrium and left ventricle, is the most vulnerable to damage, followed by the aortic valve, which controls blood flow from the left ventricle into the aorta. The triple-leaflet tricuspid valve, between the upper and lower chambers on the right side of the heart, usually escapes direct damage, but it may fail under the strain of increased back pressure transmitted through the pulmonary arteries from the other side of the heart as a consequence of mitral or aortic valvular damage. (The pulmonary valves themselves rarely need replacement, except in cases of congenital defects.)

Damage to heart valves produces two kinds of problems: *insufficiency*, which means the valve leaks through leaflets that are unable to close tightly, and *stenosis*, which means the valve opening is narrowed by growths, scars or abnormal deposits on the leaflets. Elements of insufficiency and stenosis are often present in a single damaged valve. When a valve fails to close properly, some of the blood that is pumped through it regurgitates or leaks, and the chamber that was supposed to have emptied during the contraction of systole partially fills instead with the same blood it had pumped out. This, in turn, eventually causes blood to back up in the lungs, where the increased pressure leads to pulmonary edema.

To accommodate the abnormal flow of blood from the aorta back into the left ventricle, in the case of aortic insufficiency, or back into the left atrium, in the case of mitral insufficiency, the heart works harder. But the extra cardiac effort exacts a toll over a period of years, and the heart successively enlarges, weakens and goes into failure. The same sequence occurs when a narrowed opening restricts the normal flow of blood into the left ventricle, in the case of mitral stenosis, or into the aorta, in the case of aortic stenosis.

In its early symptomatic stages, cardiac valvular disease causes a person to become easily fatigued. Then, as the stenosis or insufficiency progresses, the main symptom of heart failure—breathlessness—appears. Without surgery or medical drug therapy, the condition will only worsen, deepening into acute or chronic heart failure and, frequently, setting off such arrhythmias as atrial fibrillation in which the top chambers beat irregularly and much faster than the lower ones (decreasing the heart's output by 15 to 25 percent). Another danger is the possible formation of a blood clot in the atrium as a consequence of sluggish blood flow. The clot, if it is large enough to block the valve and prevent passage of blood into the ventricle, can cause fainting, or if it is not dislodged by natural turbulence within the chamber, it can prove fatal. The clot may shed smaller particles that pass through the valve and lodge in small vessels, perhaps in a kidney, where it blocks circulation and destroys tissue, or in the brain, where similar effects cause the condition familiarly known as a stroke.

The body's normal immunological defense against certain bacteria, particularly those responsible for strep throat, can trigger a damaging reaction in the mitral and, less often, in the aortic valves, causing, years after the initial infection, the condition known as rheumatic heart disease, in which the affected valve leaflets are thickened and often fused along their edges. The initial infection, which may lead to rheumatic heart disease, is caused by streptococcal bacteria. When they invade the body, these organisms often produce a disease known simply as rheumatic fever, which lasts for about two weeks. During this time, joints, especially those in the knees and ankles, may become painful and swollen, the back of the throat often becomes red and sore, and the lining of the interior of the heart may become inflamed. Not everyone who contracts rheumatic fever, however, develops all these symptoms. Sometimes the disease does not affect the heart at all. But when it does, researchers believe that the lasting damage results from an overreaction of the body's immunological system to the invading bacteria that settle on the heart's valves. Over a period of years, sometimes as long as twenty years after the initial infection, the valve leaflets may become thickened with calcium deposits and fibrous tissue—the same kind of tissue that forms in a scar. In the last two or three decades, the aggressive use of specific antibiotics in the treatment of strep throat has effectively pushed rheumatic fever from first place as the cause of valvular damage in the United States, and now the leading causes of valvular damage are degenerative changes produced by aging; heart attacks that injure the mitral valve's papillary muscles, which normally close the valve tightly after each heartbeat; and certain bacteria that invade the bloodstream and settle on valve leaflets that have been made susceptible by previous injury.

Since 1962, when valves damaged beyond repair were first successfully replaced, many types of artificial substitutes have been developed. The porcine valve—a specially processed valve from the heart of a pig—developed in France by Alan Carpentier, M.D., and first used in 1970, has become increasingly popular as a replacement for damaged valves in an adult heart. Unlike transplanted human valves, which are known as homograft valves and are taken from cadavers, the porcine valve is not living tissue. If it were, it would be rejected as foreign by the body's immunological system. Instead, the cells are rendered inert by a chemical such as glutaraldehyde, which "tans" the valve somewhat as leather is tanned. The valve retains its strength and flexibility even though the tissue is no longer alive, and according to its advocates, it comes closer to matching the flow characteristics of the natural human valve (pigs and humans have remarkably similar hearts) than do most mechanical valves.

Nevertheless, many surgeons still prefer to use a modified, cloth-covered version of the silicone rubber ball-in-a-cage valve developed by Albert Starr, M.D., and M.L. Edwards, M.D., at the University of Oregon. The ball floats freely in its cage to permit blood to pass from atrium to ventricle or ventricle to aorta, but when the blood attempts to reverse its flow, the ball jams tightly against the opening and stops it. In some instances the function of the natural valve itself can be restored with a ring prosthesis called the Cooley ring, or C-ring, after its developer, Denton A. Cooley, M.D., of the Texas Heart Institute. The device, which is actually a semicircle of flexible Dacron tape covered with Dacron velour, is placed, like a collar, around the floppy, ballooned-out leaflets of a damaged valve to help it shut properly.

The surgical insertion of an artificial valve—which, considering hospital and surgical fees, can cost around $20,000—involves risks, as many other heart operations do, that depend on such factors as the patient's physical condition and age; associated diseases such as diabetes, hypertension and coronary artery disease; and the degree of damage that the valvular condition has already produced in the heart. These need to be evaluated against the risks of not having surgery. There are also long-term risks after the operation:

- Bacteria may lodge on the surface of the artificial valve—which, unlike normal tissue, has no germ-killing qualities—and spread to the normal heart tissue, where they can cause endocarditis, an infection of the heart's lining. For this reason, valve patients need special antibiotic therapy as a precaution during illnesses and before any additional surgery, even before a procedure as minor as a tooth extraction.
- Blood clots are also a continuing hazard for valve recipients, occurring at the rate of 2 to 3 percent a year for aortic valve replacements and 5 percent a year for mitral valves. All patients

with mechanical valves are required therefore to take anticoagulant medication daily for the rest of their lives, and antiplatelet medication on occasion. (Anticoagulants are usually not required for patients with animal-tissue valves.)

• Unnatural blood turbulence around the mechanical valves can damage red blood cells, causing anemia. This condition can easily be diagnosed after an appropriate blood test, and iron tablets can correct it.

• The valve itself is subject to wear and dysfunction. But if trouble develops, it usually happens gradually, leaving ample time to replace the valve with a new one.

At this writing, none of the available artificial heart valves can be considered permanent replacements. They have a maximum life, on average, of ten years. However, improvements are continually being made, and it is expected that newer versions, which are undergoing careful laboratory tests, will function significantly longer with fewer side effects when they are perfected for human use.

Despite the drawbacks, which are actually quite minor considering the alternative of having no suitable substitute at all, the artificial valves offer more than just a new gateway for blood to flow through the heart. They offer a new gateway to life for people whose damaged natural valves make living nearly impossible.

19

HEART TRANSPLANT: THE LAST RESORT

In the late summer of 1977, death seemed appallingly near for William Hougesen as he lay in bed in Chicago's St. Joseph's Hospital, weakened to the point that he could barely raise his head. He was trying, without much luck, to recover from his third heart attack in as many years and from a rapidly progressing condition known as cardiomyopathy in which cardiac muscle—perhaps because of a viral or bacterial infection—begins degenerating. His heart, in the words of his doctor, had stretched and enlarged like an old balloon that has been inflated a long time. Its resiliency was gone and its pumping action was deteriorating day after day.

Nothing the doctors tried seemed to help, and one Sunday morning, hours after two consulting cardiologists confirmed that further treatment would be fruitless, Hougesen's personal physician stopped by his patient's room with an unusual request: Would he please watch a specific television program that night?

The show, a *Nova* documentary, described the heart-transplantation program at Stanford University Medical Center in Palo Alto, California, the only such program in the United States at the time. On Monday morning, in response to his doctor's question about his thoughts on the *Nova* show, Hougesen smiled wryly and said that he felt sorry "for any poor devil who has to be subjected to that." It was not the response his doctor was anticipating, but Hougesen's sentiments can be excused because he had not yet realized—as he would over the next few days—that heart transplantation was his last hope and that Stanford University Medical Center would be his next stop, if after tests he was found to be a suitable candidate for the dramatic life-saving operation.

It was at Stanford in 1959 that Norman E. Shumway, M.D., and his colleagues performed the first animal heart transplant in a dog and developed the technique used by South Africa's Christiaan Barnard, M.D., when he performed the world's first successful transplantation of a human heart on December 3, 1967. The Stanford team, headed by Dr. Shumway, performed the second human heart transplantation in the United States, the fourth in the world, little more than a month later, on January 6, 1968, and during that year, 101 heart transplants were done by sixty-four surgical teams in twenty-two countries in a burst of surgical enthusiasm fanned by wide and heady publicity. Within a year or two, that enthusiasm waned as surgeons, sobered by the reality that almost all of their heart-transplant patients died within a year of the operation, abandoned the procedure. Some, including Dr. Shumway, however, quietly persisted with the operation, concentrating their efforts on counteracting the body's rejection of the transplanted heart, which had accounted for the dismal failure rate.

Since 1968, the Stanford heart-transplant team has done over 180 operations; over 70 of their patients are still alive, some after having a second and even a third new heart. The one-year survival rate among the Stanford patients has increased from 22 percent to 69 percent, and the five-year survival rate, which is about 50 percent, rivals that of kidney transplantation. It has been a stunning comeback for an operation that was faltering not because of inadequate surgical technique, but because of the natural phenomenon of rejection, a phenomenon that can now be detected in its early development and thwarted with appropriate medication.

Even in the light of the recent impressive survival rates, heart transplantation is still fraught with risks, and to make sure that a patient has every chance of surviving, the hospital has to make an enormous commitment in resources and manpower to prepare not only for the operation itself but also for the postoperative consequences of rejection. In the handful of hospitals around the country where the operation is still undertaken—led by Stanford, where one half of the world's heart transplants have been done— the patients are selected with painstaking care. Only one in five who applies to Stanford's heart transplant program passes the initial screening, which is based primarily on information furnished by the patient's regular physician.

On September 7, 1977, Bill Hougesen learned that he was among the lucky one-fifth, the first fortuitous news he had after a long series of setbacks in his fight against heart disease. He and his wife, Maria, flew to Stanford for the final four-day physical and psychological evaluation. Stanford doctors found Hougesen to be an ideal candidate for a new heart. He did not have any of the chronic diseases—such as diabetes, hypertension, kidney disease or advanced pulmonary congestion—which disqualify so many potential heart-transplant recipients. Apart from his damaged heart, Bill Hougesen's body was as healthy as that of any other forty-eight-year-old who has led a relatively active life, and he was optimistic and willing to face the demanding days ahead of him. On September 12 he was told that he had passed the final screening and had been accepted into the program. Now came the wait for a suitable donor heart.

Life expectancy for those accepted into the Stanford program is measured in weeks or months, and for some, the time runs out before a donor heart can be found. The average wait is thirty-three days—but some wait much longer. Of 32 qualified candidates in the Stanford program who died before a new heart could be found, 30 survived twenty-one weeks or less.

As they were advised, Hougesen and his wife rented an apartment close to the hospital, and the agony of the calendar began. Waiting for his new heart, Bill Hougesen recalls, was the worst experience of his life. He was very weak and suffering so much that he was unable to describe how bad he felt. He was, in his wife's words, literally slipping away.

On visits to the medical center for checkups, Bill became acquainted with others also camped out in motels and apartments near the hospital awaiting new hearts. One fortunate young woman who was suffering from cardiomyopathy (the heart condition that accounts for 40 percent of the transplants at Stanford) received a matching heart as soon as she arrived in Palo Alto. Another patient, a young boy from Europe, arrived to find a suitable heart waiting for him, but he was temporarily disqualified because he was running a slight fever, a symptom of a possible infection that could have endangered the transplant. The heart went to another young patient, and when another heart finally became available, the operation was too late. He died a few days after surgery.

At 12:30 A.M. on October 27, after seven weeks of thinking that it was the hospital calling every time the phone rang, Hougesen got "the call." The donor heart would come from a young man whose skull had been crushed in a motorcycle accident, but whose organs were still functioning as he lay, hooked up to a mechanical respirator, in a nearby hospital. Three independent consultants had confirmed the diagnosis of "brain death" as evidenced by the absence of electrical activity in the brain. After permission had been obtained from the victim's relatives, the body, with a portable respirator pumping air into the lungs, was rushed by ambulance to Stanford, where the heart-transplant team was assembling, and tests which showed that the donor heart would match well with Hougesen's tissues were done.

If heart transplantation were only a matter of good surgery, all those who have received new hearts, according to Dr. Shumway, would live. The problem is that the body of a person who has received a new heart perceives the new tissue to be foreign material to be attacked and rejected by the body's natural defense system—just as it rejects an invasion of bacteria or even a splinter under the skin. The doctors expected Hougesen's body to start rejecting the new heart as soon as it was implanted. But if the match was a good one—as tests showed it would be—the reaction could be managed by drugs that suppress the body's immune system.

A good match involves not only the pairing of donor and recipient by blood type—A, B, AB or O—but also the pairing of the respective organs by tissue type, a newer classification of inherited substances that make organs uniquely or nearly uniquely individual. Tissue types are the internal equivalent of fingerprints. There are many more tissue types than blood types, which makes it considerably more difficult to obtain a match. For a transplanted organ—no matter whether it is a kidney or a heart—to be compatible (that is, not to be rejected), preliminary tests have to be made on cells called lymphocytes, which carry on their surfaces the same antigens or tissue type as do organs. A good match means that a number of these surface factors from the donor and recipient are identical. The best matches are between identical twins—and after that among family members. Sometimes good matches can come from unrelated people, but that is a matter of chance, as Hougesen found out.

Also affecting the chances for rejection are the presence of antibodies in the donated organ or in the recipient, created years earlier by the body's immune defenses against specific diseases such as mumps or measles. Thus, there are thousands of possible substances lurking in a person's bloodstream or on the surface of his tissues which can foster rejection, and even a match between identical twins may not be perfect.

Of all the potential recipients on Stanford's heart-transplant waiting list the morning of October 27, the tissue type of the heart of the motorcyclist came closest to matching the tissue type of Hougesen's heart. The long wait was over, and as Bill Hougesen lay in a partly anesthetized daze on the operating table the thought occurred to him that this is "probably the end, but at least it will be without any more pain—not a bad way to go."

In the Shumway heart-transplant technique, blood is kept from entering the heart by tying off the two large veins feeding the right atrium and by clamping the aorta to prevent backflow. The recipient's circulation is then diverted into a heart-lung machine, where it is oxygenated before being pumped back into a major artery. The fibrous sac surrounding the now stilled heart is opened with a lengthwise incision, and its edges are stitched to the opened chest wall to form a basin, or as Dr. Shumway calls it, a pericardial cradle, into which near-freezing saline solution will be introduced to chill and preserve the new heart during the thirty-five-minute period when it does not beat.

Instead of severing and tediously reconnecting the two large veins supplying the right atrium and the four pulmonary veins entering the left atrium of Bill Hougesen's heart, one of the surgeons on the heart-transplant team made an incision through the atria, leaving the top section of each chamber in place. Next he severed the two great vessels which empty the heart—the pulmonary trunk and the aorta—and lifted the swollen, diseased heart out of Bill Hougesen's chest.

For a moment Hougesen lay on the table with only a cavity

where his heart had been. Then the surgeon who had removed the donor heart in an adjacent operating room carried the organ, lying in a bowl of chilled saline, a few steps to his waiting colleagues. The new heart was eased into position, stilled and stitched to matching segments of the remaining, old atria. When it was finally secured in place, it was flushed out with cold saline, and then, as the clamps holding back Hougeson's circulation were removed, it swelled with blood. After a brief electrical jolt, it began a strong beat.

Essentially, the operation was over, and more important, a success. But for safety's sake, the surgeons delayed closure for nearly forty-five minutes as they watched for leaks or any abnormalities. When all seemed well, they closed the chest, and Bill Hougesen was moved into his own private intensive care unit. The entire procedure had taken four hours.

His continued survival, however, was dependent on his doctor's ability to prevent his body from rejecting its borrowed heart. The dreaded event, known as a rejection crisis—which begins when the body's white blood cells invade and destroy heart tissue—can be diagnosed by electrocardiograms and blood tests, but neither of these methods is as sensitive as a test developed in 1972 in which a doctor inserts a narrow tubular device with a clipper on the end through the jugular vein in the neck and into the heart, where the jaws of the clipper retrieve a snippet of heart muscle for microscopic analysis.

Twelve times Bill Hougesen underwent this minute biopsy of his heart, performed under local anesthetic, and three times the analysis indicated that his body had begun to reject its new heart. Hougesen's dosages of immunosuppressive drugs were increased and a powerful drug known as antithymocyte globulin (ATG)—a factor artificially produced in the blood of rabbits—was injected to counter the destructive action of the white blood cells on the donor heart.

Bill Hougesen was sequestered in a $400-a-day private room behind double doors and an antechamber. Around the clock a private nurse guarded him from nonessential intrusions by staff members and recleaned the room and its utensils with disinfectants whenever a necessary visitor stopped by. Anyone who entered the room was required to wear a surgical mask, rubber gloves and an over-the-clothing gown, as did Bill when he ventured out of his room for daily physical therapy in the hospital gymnasium.

Patients previously noted for their good humor frequently become sullen and demanding during the recovery period, a side effect of the medication, which in Bill Hougesen's case caused him to awaken some mornings with "indescribable feelings of terror" that plunged him into depression. The nurses warned his wife that such mood changes might occur, and she agrees that he was at times difficult during his seventy-seven days in the hospital. On his release from the hospital in early January he was advised to remain in the rented apartment with his wife so that he could visit the medical center for twice-weekly checkups, during which x-ray photographs were taken of his heart. Tantalum coils, inserted in his heart during surgery, showed up in the x-rays and helped his doctors to assess how well his heart was responding to exercise and the rejection-combating drugs.

On February 20, 1978, after five and a half months in California, the Hougesens were told that they could return home to Chicago. Bill, who had been a commanding officer with the rank of captain in the police communications center, was reassigned to head the medical unit at the police training academy, where he would oversee the physical fitness, health and physical examinations of recruits. Within two years of his return, he was qualified by the police surgeon to perform any kind of police duty, behind a desk or in the field.

His personal exercise program, which had begun moderately, was expanded to include a daily four-mile walk at a pace brisk enough for him to complete the walk in one hour. Three days a week at the police training academy, he joins a gym class where he has steadily increased his performance until, at this writing, he is able to do 50 push-ups, 200 sit-ups and 150 "leg-overs" in the course of the exercise period. He tried jogging a few times, but after a quarter of a mile his breathing became labored and his throat and lungs burned. This might sound like a contradiction for a man supposedly in good physical condition, but the trouble, he knew, lay in the fact that no nerves connect his new heart to his brain. Such nerve reconnection is not possible in a transplant. Hougesen cannot feel his heart—nor would he feel a heart attack if he happened to have one. If he runs or is startled or excited, his heart begins to beat more rapidly, but after a delay, not instantaneously as when nerves signal the heart to leap into action. Hougesen's heart accelerates only after adrenalin and other hormone stimulants have had time to travel from the secreting glands via the bloodstream to the heart.

Every day for the remainder of his life, Hougesen will be reminded of the debt he owes to medical science by the unavoidable fact that he has to take 37 pills, some to prevent rejection, some to supplement the body's defenses, and still others to offset the side effects of the first two categories. It is something he has to live with. The process by which the coronary arteries of his new heart may become clogged with plaques is stimulated by his own body's reaction to the new tissue, and it can be accelerated by a rich diet. Thus, the emphasis on low-cholesterol diet.

Pill number 38 is a prospect which Hougesen knows he will face. Pills 39 and 40, and even others, may be added to his medication regimen as researchers develop better ways to combat rejection. The thirty-eighth pill, for which Hougesen is a candidate, is an antiplatelet drug that has been found to interfere with plaque formation and at the same time diminishes the need for immunosuppressants. The medication has already proved successful in protecting some heart-attack patients from subsequent heart damage.

As the phenomenon of rejection yields its secrets and as more and more is learned about the body's immune defenses against a transplanted heart, the therapy designed to keep a new heart functioning will unquestionably improve. Nevertheless, heart transplantation is only a limited solution, dependent as it is on the availability of a suitable donor heart; when no heart is available, it is not a solution at all. The ultimate solution to the disorders that cripple the human heart lies in the hands of researchers who are developing the artificial heart, as well as in the hands of other investigators who are patiently unraveling the puzzling abnormalities that still plague the heart. Of course, for patients like Bill Hougesen, there is no perfected artificial alternative to a healthy donor heart, and time is not on their side. For them, heart transplantation, despite a price tag of $40,000 for the operation and hospitalization and $2,500 for medication and tests each year afterward, is their best—and only—hope for staying alive.

20

THE ARTIFICIAL HEART

The red-painted brick façade of Old St. Mark's Hospital looms up amid the high grass a few blocks from the northwest edge of Salt Lake City and the beginning of the desert. It is a fairly anonymous place—some city cabdrivers claim never to have heard of it—and from a distance it is easy to see why, for the hospital appears long abandoned, and in a way it is. The building no longer can lay claim to being—in the strict sense of the word—a hospital. Its front wing has been given over to a prison rehabilitation clinic, and around back, past blocked-off entrances that reinforce the sense of the building's lost past, is a nondescript rear door, a portal, if you will, that opens onto the anticipatory, quiet fervor of scientists actively engaged in perfecting the world's best hope for one eventual solution to cardiac disease: the artificial heart.

It is here in these unlikely surroundings that Willem J. Kolff, M.D., Ph.D., a Dutch-born inventive genius, has set up his laboratories under the auspices of the University of Utah's Division of Artificial Organs, which he has headed since being lured to the university in 1967 from a similar position at the Cleveland Clinic. Dr. Kolff, whose landmark achievements stretch back to the early 1940s when he invented the artificial kidney, and include important developments in the creation of the heart-lung machine and cardiac-assist devices, has assembled a close-knit team of physicians, engineers, chemists and technicians to help him build an array of artificial organs that could eventually bring the *Six Million Dollar Man* out of the realm of fiction.

Emanating from a room at the rear of the first floor, an aroma not unlike that of a barn permeates the entranceway. Those in the know regard it as olfactory proof of the laboratory's success so far in developing the long-promised artificial heart for man. Three black-and-white Holstein calves stabled in the back room and responsible for the unexpected olfactory stimulant in the air are being kept alive by a trio of air-powered polyurethane hearts designed by Robert Jarvik, M.D., a staff scientist on the Kolff team with a background in zoology and bioengineering. Air hoses connected to the internal pumps lead out of the animals' bodies to consoles above the three steel cages, which control the artificial hearts. Other tubes and wires connect to a bank of computers along the opposite wall to monitor the hearts and record data. It was here that a retired sixty-one-year-old Seattle dentist by the name of Barney Clark came to view the artificial heart in action and to make a crucial decision that would lead him to become the world's first human recipient of the plastic and aluminum heart known as the Jarvik-7.

Until Dr. Clark's chest was opened and his worn-out heart was replaced with the Jarvik-7, the world's record for survival with an artificial heart was held by a calf named Lord Tennyson. The black-and-white Holstein lived 268 days with an earlier model—the Jarvik-5—artificial heart. The experiments with animals and artificial hearts, which Dr. Kolff began in 1957, paved the way for the first human implantation late in 1982.

The quest for an artificial heart has been riddled with failure and disappointing setbacks since the late 1960s and early 1970s when the feats of biomedical engineering that had produced artificial blood vessels, pacemakers and mechanical heart valves seemed to be on the verge of producing the artificial heart itself. That expectation turned out to be vastly premature, and the artificial-heart program, which started out with millions of dollars in federal support and glowing engineering assessments, faltered badly. Controversy not only enveloped the social and ethical implications of the nascent technology ("Who will get the first artificial heart?" "Will it unmercifully prolong life in hopeless cases?") but it also conflicted with the then Atomic Energy Commission's efforts to harness nuclear energy to run the artificial heart. At stake was the development of a plutonium pellet that had been widely heralded as the fuel for the artificial pump's thermal engine. As it turned out, this novel approach has been largely abandoned.

In the period of retrenchment that followed these unsettling times, many of the leading artificial-heart researchers went back to their laboratories to rethink "the problem with more humility toward God's handiwork," according to one critic of the heart program, quoted by the New York *Times*. The problems inherent in the design and construction of a clinically practical artificial heart are imposing, to say the least. The building material must not harm the blood (by abrading the delicate red blood cells or initiating the process of clot formation), as even the most gentle of synthetic substances seem to do after a time. Nor must it create clots, which can travel through the bloodstream and lodge with destructive consequences in such organs as the brain or lungs. At the same time, the material must be resilient enough to expand and contract 60 to 100 times a minute, twenty-four hours a day, day in, day out, for years.

The technology to this end culminated in the development of a heart fashioned from polyurethane plastic and surgical-grade aluminum and driven to pump by air forced through tubes from a compressor. The Jarvik-7 is a marvel of technology. In place of cardiac muscle, it has a four-layered polyurethane diaphragm, each layer separated by a dry graphite lubricant. The diaphragm responds by bulging upward to push the blood through the rigid heart and out through the natural blood vessels to which it is attached.

To keep the blood flowing in the proper direction, polycarbonate rings support tilting-disk valves that open and shut in response to pressures inside the heart. Surrounding each of the four valves —two for each of the separate left and right artificial ventricles— are Dacron mesh cuffs that are sewn on to the patient's natural atria. The cuff and the artificial ventricles are equipped with snaps that allow them to be attached to each other. And the ventricles themselves are secured to each other by Velcro fabric fasteners. The whole arrangement allows for replacement of individual parts in case of a malfunction.

Efforts to develop an artificial heart followed several paths. The most promising of these has been the development of the left ventricular assist device (LVAD), which is not a whole artificial heart, but rather half of one. Such devices are valuable adjuncts in helping an ailing heart recover after surgery, for instance to replace a valve, until the heart has regained strength enough to pump sufficiently on its own. Most of the federal funding is being funneled to research programs where the emphasis is on such devices, which are under development at eleven centers in the United States, including the University of Utah, as well as at research centers in Germany, Japan, Austria and Switzerland.

The first successful use of a heart-assist device dates back to the late 1960s when partially implantable models were used temporarily in cardiac-surgery patients who could not be weaned from the heart-lung machine because once restarted, their hearts beat too feebly. The heart-lung machine, for all its value, can maintain a patient for only five hours or so before it damages too many blood cells and begins causing clots. If the heart is not strong enough to pump effectively on its own after that time limit, surgeons can use a heart-assist device known as an intraortic balloon pump; it was conceived in 1961 by Dr. Kolff's group and perfected six years later by Adrian Kantrowitz, M.D., then at Maimonides Medical Center in Brooklyn, and now associated with Sinai Hospital of Detroit. The device, which boosts a faint heartbeat by inflating and deflating a narrow balloon that is inserted into the aorta, not only permits surgeons to disconnect the heart-lung machine without fatal consequences but also allows the heart time to recover if it is going to.

The newer, fully implantable LVADs with self-contained power sources are designed, though still experimental, to take over the work of the left ventricle—as the name implies—from the seemingly improbable albeit roomy implantation site in the abdominal cavity. Large tubes will ascend from the LVAD to draw blood out of the left atrium or ventricle and carry it back into the circulation via the aorta after a slight detour in the artificial pumping chamber of the LVAD. One such device, being built and tested by Andros, Inc., of Berkeley, California, under the direction of its research chief, Peer M. Portner, Ph.D., employs a seamless sac, dual-pusher plate blood pump, integrated into a single motorized unit that is controlled by a microcomputer powered by re-chargeable nickel-cadmium batteries.

The Kolff team's entry into the LVAD field is based on half of the artificial heart. Actually, the Jarvik artificial heart, which is deceptively simple, is not a replacement for the entire heart. It consists only of the lower chambers, which, in most cases, can be sutured to the natural upper chambers that are rarely damaged in heart failure. The artificial chambers themselves are about the size and shape of a normal heart's ventricles and they weigh about the same as a normal, healthy heart—280 grams.

Surgery to implant the first Jarvik-7 into a human being began several hours ahead of schedule late on the night of December 1, 1982, when Dr. Clark was rushed into surgery because his own heart was about to give out. Clark had been suffering from a trio of heart ailments that, it had been speculated, began with a myste-rious viral infection that led to an inflammation of his heart mus-cle. His condition deteriorated over four years as progressive amounts of his heart grew inflamed and died, to be replaced by scar tissue that is ineffectual in helping the heart beat strongly.

Scars, combined with progressive inflammation, caused Clark's heart to fail gradually. Because he was too old for a transplant, and drugs no longer could help, Clark opted to become the first recipi-ent of the artificial heart. After meeting all the requirements set by the University of Utah and the Food and Drug Administration, which regulates medical devices, the only thing he could look forward to was dying, according to the surgeon who performed the implant, William DeVries, M.D., chairman of cardiovascular and thoracic surgery at the University of Utah Medical Center.

Early in the morning of December 2, 1982—one day short of the fifteenth anniversary of the first human heart transplantation—Dr. DeVries was handed a blue sterile cloth under which, according to the label, was the "Total Artificial Heart No. 1 with percutane-ous leads." The leads would, hours later, be connected to a mobile control unit the size of a portable television, and at 6:20 A.M. EST, Barney Clark began living on the Jarvik-7, tethered by six feet of hose to air compressors that empower the rhythmic pumping to circulate his blood. He lived with the artificial heart for 112 days. In March 1983, Barney Clark died of circulatory collapse following multiple organ system failure.

The next major stage in the Kolff team's vision of the artificial heart is a miniature, built-in electric motor to replace the air compressor—a technological advancement that is based on the giant pulsating engine used on icebreakers to move fluid ballast from one side of the ship to the other. The brushless DC motor, according to the engineers designing it, will be about the size and shape of a lipstick. A tiny turbine on the end of the rotor shaft will be capable of reversing the flow of hydraulic fluid (probably water) running through it, alternately compressing the artificial ventricles and thereby duplicating the pumping action of the natural heart. The motor could be powered from a four- to five-pound compact, wearable nickel-cadmium battery pack that could be recharged with regular household electricity during the day or alternatively at night by an electrically charged induction coil built into a special mattress which would transmit electricity to an induction coil worn by the artificial-heart recipient during sleep. A stand-by battery pack and electronic controls could be implanted just under the skin (probably at the waist) for emergencies when the main power source fails or unexpectedly runs down. Plans call for a microcomputer, about the size of a pack of playing cards, to be built into the energy packs to regulate the beat according to the body's needs. It will accelerate the artificial heart when the wearer runs or otherwise undergoes exertion and will slow down during rest, just as the natural heart does.

In the far future an artificial heart may, according to the Utah group's speculation, be powered by the oxidation of blood glucose —the source of power for the natural heart.

The basic polyurethane ventricles, which can be mass-produced from molds, should cost less than $1,000, and the electric motor with its control unit should only add another $200, according to Steven Nielsen, the University of Utah electrical engineer who is developing the circuitry and perfecting the motor. The surgery to implant the artificial heart and the hospitalization afterward should be far less costly than that of a heart transplant because, according to the Kolff team's estimates, most of the cost of a heart transplant involves months of fighting the body's effort to reject the transplanted heart, the beginning of a lifelong process. This is not necessary with the artificial heart, for the body does not try to reject it.

Estimates of the number of people who might benefit from an artificial heart vary from a low of 17,000 annually, according to figures derived by the NHLBI several years ago, to a high of 160,000, according to the Stanford Research Institute.

As expected, enormous public interest—as well as the attendant controversy—arose after the artificial heart moved from the laboratory into actual clinical use. Discussion moved from the theoretical arena to practical considerations such as who would be chosen to receive an artificial heart. Would it be people who could afford it? (Clark's artificial heart and the attending efforts of those who implanted it were donated.) Who would pay for it otherwise?

There have been other advances in heart surgery that have been dependent on mechanical devices, and these have entered the health-care arena without undue controversy. Perhaps the pace at which the artificial heart is being developed, with interim stages such as the left ventricular assist device, will give needed breathing space, so to speak, so that our society can come to grips with the ethical, moral, psychological, economic and legal problems that a totally implantable artificial heart poses. For instance, who would be chosen to receive the first one? Would it be the person who could afford it? Who would pay for it otherwise? If the artificial heart kept pumping, would the recipient technically "live" forever? What criteria would be used to pronounce death?

A few years ago Dr. Kolff and other experts from many fields sat down at a conference in Washington, D.C., to discuss just these implications. Very little was resolved, but the important point is that concerned men and women met to exchange views about a future technology that they knew would have a vast impact when it eventually arrives. Rather than have the technology unwittingly unleashed and accept the consequences and deal with the problem after the fact, they were willing and able to start what in the language of the day was called "a dialogue." Those efforts have continued, taken up by other people in other places.

One must recognize that the complex moral and economic factors make it unlikely that discussion of their significance will ever end.

21

THE SEARCH FOR SOLUTIONS

Mindful that the business of making predictions about the outcome of medical research entails the risk of being wrong, the Cleveland Clinic's Irvine H. Page, M.D., cautioned that when a breakthrough does come, it could be from a direction we least expect. Yet, surely, glimpses of the future can be obtained by examining all three fronts (the diagnosis of coronary heart disease, its treatment and prevention) where research has paved the way for notable triumphs that may mark this decade as the final turning point in the battle against heart disease.

The Rapid Heart-Attack Test

In many cases a heart attack is not obvious, either to the person who has suffered it or to the physician who is trying to detect its telltale evidence. Indeed, most people in coronary intensive care units have not suffered a heart attack; they are there because their doctors suspect they may have had a heart attack. But even the experts have to wait two or three days for the results of conclusive enzyme tests that detect the presence of substances released by dying heart muscle cells.

That situation is changing, thanks to the work of two young cardiologists who, building on the work of researchers before them, have devised a heart attack detection test that cuts the waiting time to less than two hours. Michael H. Burnham, M.D., and

William E. Shell, M.D., both at Cedars-Sinai Hospital in Los Angeles and associate professors of cardiology at the University of California at Los Angeles, spent a year and a half and analyzed 700 patients in the course of their discovery. If it proves as successful in widespread testing as it was at Cedars-Sinai, it may revolutionize heart care, save tens or even hundreds of millions of dollars a year in coronary intensive care unit costs, and spare thousands of patients needless anxiety. Each year, according to figures derived from insurance-company studies, some 250,000 Americans who have suspected heart attacks and have been cared for in CCUs turn out to have had false alarms.

The Burnham and Shell test not only gives far quicker results but is also far more accurate than the standard test, which fails to detect some heart attacks and, in other instances, sometimes falsely indicates that they have occurred in healthy people.

Both tests are based on an analysis of blood samples for specific enzymes that are released into the circulation by heart cells that die during a heart attack. The serial enzyme test (so called because several tests are made over two or three days) could not distinguish between enzymes released by dying brain cells or dying skeletal muscle cells and those released by dying heart tissue. Drs. Burnham and Shell, however, found a way to manufacture an antibody that attaches to the heart-enzyme fraction only. The antibody is tagged with a radioactive tracer, and the resulting radioactivity of the blood sample is measured to detect the presence of the specific heart enzyme.

Dr. Burnham believes that the greatest benefit of the rapid, supersensitive test will be in identifying heart-attack victims within hours rather than days after they come to the hospital.

A CAT Scanner for the Heart

The machine itself is as imposing in appearance as it is in performance. The patient lies supine at the core of a giant cylinder, surrounded by a rotating framework holding twenty-eight x-ray tubes, which whirl around him in a complete revolution every four seconds. A descendant of the CAT scanner (computerized axial tomography), the intricate fifteen-ton diagnostic instrument provides never-before-seen views of the anatomy of the beating heart and the circulation of blood through its arteries.

The traditional CAT scanner, which has revolutionized diagnosis in some areas of the body, particularly in the brain, was of little value when it came to analyzing motion of the beating heart or the circulating blood. Each picture took a full second, during which there could be no motion, and only one cross section, rather than the whole organ, could be recorded at a time. To adapt it to capture images of the moving heart, investigators at the Mayo Foundation and Clinic in Rochester, Minnesota, devised a system that takes hundreds of multiple-angle x-ray images of the beating heart within a second and transmits them to image-intensifying video cameras connected to the memory bank of a computer. As the x-ray sources click on and off, views of the patient's heart are formed on a semicircular fluorescent screen. The final result is the beating heart in three-dimensional action. With appropriate computer commands, the examining physician can look at the living organ slice by slice from top to bottom or side to side. Any areas of heart muscle that are not functioning, any vessels that are obstructed, any valve that is not opening or shutting fully will show up on the fluorescent screen, aiding the physician in his diagnosis and pinpointing the trouble for surgeons. The function of the heart after corrective measures are taken can also be assessed.

Descendants of the Mayo team's machine, which are expected to cost about $2 million (four times as much as a CAT scanner), will probably be in general use in major medical centers in the late 1980s.

Nuclear Imaging

Low-dosage, short-lived radioactive material which is injected into a patient's vein is helping physicians detect coronary heart disease long before angina pectoris gives its warning. If an ordinary electrocardiogram has alerted a physician to a possible heart problem in one of his patients or if a family history of coronary artery disease plus other risk factors are positive, a nuclear-imaging test will spotlight areas of insufficient oxygen in the heart if they are present. In the test, radioactive material, such as thallium-

201, travels through the bloodstream to the heart, where gamma rays that it emits are picked up by a scintillation camera and transformed by computer into a video display of the heart, showing perfusion of the heart muscle supplied by the coronary arteries. Distribution of blood throughout the heart may appear uniform at first while the suspected heart-disease victim is at rest. But the video picture taken during an exercise stress test, when the heart needs more oxygen, may show dark spots indicative of starved heart muscle. The probable cause is a coronary artery that is narrowed enough to diminish the blood supply to a portion of the heart, but not yet blocked enough to cause angina.

Alternatives to Bypass

The bypass operation (see Chapter 17, "The Bypass") has been the dominant heart operation since the 1970s. But it is costly, drastic and not always a long-term success. Can some simpler technique replace it?

The answer, in some cases, may lie in a bold procedure with the cumbersome name of percutaneous transluminal coronary angioplasty (PTCA). Developed by Andreas R. Gruntzig, M.D., director of Interventional Cardiovascular Medicine at Emory University Hospital, Atlanta, Georgia, the technique is utterly simple and direct. A balloon-tipped catheter is threaded into a coronary artery narrowed by atherosclerosis. When the balloon reaches the narrowed portion of the artery it is inflated, and the expansion compresses the mushy plaque against the sides of the vessel, minimizing the blockage. When the catheter is withdrawn, the squashed plaque remains compressed. Normal blood flow is restored.

Dr. Gruntzig estimates that 10 to 15 percent of the patients now undergoing bypass procedures could be treated effectively with angioplasty far less expensively. The ideal candidate for the procedure has an area of blockage in a single coronary artery and suffers from angina that cannot be relieved by medication. The potential of this new procedure is impressive and, as experience is gained, the variety of uses for the Gruntzig procedure is changing rapidly.

Dr. Gruntzig reported success in the treatment of 54 of the first 80 patients—34 his own and the rest of the patients at cooperating centers in New York City (by Simon H. Stertzer, M.D.), San Francisco (by Richard K. Myler, M.D.), and in Frankfurt, West Germany. Average narrowing among Dr. Gruntzig's own patients was reduced from 61 percent to 37 percent—good enough for normal circulation. Since Dr. Gruntzig's first report, the technique has been performed at medical centers in Philadelphia; Boston; Milwaukee; and Palo Alto, California.

In the first case in the United States, the 90-percent-occluded right coronary artery of a thirty-nine-year-old San Francisco man was opened by PTCA. Angiograms taken six months later showed continued normal blood flow through the artery. The patient felt better, could exercise more and had less angina. In many cases, according to Dr. Gruntzig, the plaque further diminishes months after the procedure through a self-healing process. Yet there are drawbacks to this alternative to bypass.

It is not useful in patients whose atherosclerotic plaques have calcified and hardened, and whose blood vessels are extremely tortuous. So far, the best results have been obtained in patients under sixty years of age who have a single well-defined obstruction in a single coronary artery. Patients who undergo the procedure have to be willing to have emergency bypass surgery if PTCA is unsuccessful and a clot or a tear occurs.

For other coronary-disease patients, including some beyond age sixty, John Simpson, M.D., of Stanford University believes the answer for safely removing, not just compressing, the obstruction is a small reaming device attached to a balloon dilating system similar to Dr. Gruntzig's. The device, which he is developing, will theoretically make a very clean cut that will remove calcium and scar tissue, as well as the soft cholesterol inside the plaque.

Dissolving the Clot

In an effort to help the thousands of Americans who suffer a heart attack, physicians try to intervene as early as possible. Since late in the spring of 1982, a drug has been available that can literally dissolve the clot that clogs a coronary artery. The drug is streptokinase, and it is delivered via a catheter directly to the coronary arteries, where it quickly—within an hour—dissolves any clotted blood that is blocking the passage through the coronary vessels.

Such treatment promises to reduce the amount of heart muscle that suffers irreparable damage from a blockage in a coronary artery and gives physicians a way to alter the course of a heart attack in progress. With the availability of streptokinase in many medical centers, it is even more important to seek emergency attention when symptoms indicate the possibility of a heart attack.

Streptokinase treatment will not replace bypass surgery; nor is it effective after heart muscle cells have died.

Shrinking the Infarct

Before long, doctors may be able to inject drugs into the heart muscle to limit the severity of heart attacks and literally shrink the area of damaged tissue. At this writing, Harvard researchers Eugene Braunwald, M.D., and Peter Hillis, M.D., are already conducting trials in humans as well as animals.

It is not that heart tissue killed in a heart attack is somehow restored to life; rather, the surrounding tissue, which is starved for oxygen and nourishment but not yet dead, is given a drug-induced boost. One infarct-limiting drug, the enzyme hyaluronidase, promotes the transport of nutrients into the blood-starved area and speeds the removal of wastes. Others that are being tested reduce the heart's work, so the damaged tissue requires less oxygen. They also increase blood flow to the damaged area by dilating collateral blood vessels.

Still another category of drugs, including steroids and cobra venom, may help the damaged heart muscle by countering inflammation and cellular disruption within the infarct.

Reversing Atherosclerosis

Robert Barndt, Jr., M.D., and David H. Blankenhorn, M.D., of the University of Southern California have shown that atherosclerosis is not necessarily an inexorable process that marches in only one direction. Over a period of thirteen months they took x-ray pictures of the leg arteries of 25 high-risk patients being treated to lower high blood cholesterol with drugs and diet. The atherosclerosis advanced in 13 patients and showed no change in 3 others. But for 9, the intensive treatment worked. Not only was the atherosclerosis stopped, but the plaques actually shrank. It is possible that the same process of plaque reduction was occurring throughout the circulatory system, including the coronary arteries.

"The experience we have obtained to date with early lesions under treatment," wrote Drs. Barndt and Blankenhorn in *Clinical Therapeutics*, "encourages us in believing that existing therapies may produce significant benefit to many persons if consistently and aggressively applied."

The best hope for the future, however, lies not in expensive technological solutions, not in fancier operations or better coronary care units, but in the elimination of the risk factors that lead to heart disease. We need to exercise more, lose weight and learn to cope better with stressful situations. We need to do this not only for ourselves, but as an example to our children. For better or worse, they emulate us. If we smoke, overeat or get too little exercise ourselves, we will lead them in the same hazardous direction.

The last quarter of a century has seen spectacular advances in our understanding of heart disease, but much mystery remains. Moreover, a "cure" for heart disease is not likely to be found; at least not in the way that the Salk and Sabin vaccines conquered polio, or penicillin vanquished some bacterial infections. Most heart disease results from several factors, rather than from the effects of a single agent.

Much of the confusion about heart disease in the public mind is due to the fragmentary way we learn about it. Each news story about an exciting research development or about a conflicting theory represents only a small view of the entire panorama. Each small controversy, each small victory becomes magnified because it is "news." If ninety-nine researchers or physicians believe one thing, and the one-hundredth loudly proclaims the opposite, he will get the headlines because he has an unusual or newsworthy view. Sometimes he is right; more often, he is not.

Contrary to the impression sometimes left by news reports, progress in heart research and treatment does not proceed at a dizzying pace, and what is learned one day is not superseded on the next. The basic rules for protecting oneself against heart disease, proclaimed two decades ago, are virtually unchanged today.

The fact that many Americans have followed these risk-factor recommendations has helped bring about the encouraging decline in heart disease over the last two decades—a decline of more than 2 percent a year.

Risk factors, even those which appear unchangeable such as age and heredity, should be a cause for action, never for despair. If your father died at age fifty of a heart attack, it does not mean you will. You simply have a better reason than the next person for consulting with your doctor and changing or eliminating any other coronary risk factors you may happen to have.

One fallacy this book has tried to correct is the idea that it is too late to change. It's never too late. But, we must remember, prevention is largely the responsibility of each of us. And the most important advice that can be given about prevention is: Begin today.

22

THE DO'S AND DON'TS OF HEART CARE

The human heart is not invincible. It is, after all, flesh and blood and subject to all the maladies that weigh upon our lives. It will beat a minimum of 40 million times a year. Over a normal lifetime, it will circulate 50 million gallons of blood. No other organ in the body shares an equal reputation for toughness and strength, for tenacity and reliability. No other organ commands quite the same philosophic and symbolic place in the ideas of man. The sound of the mother's heart is the first sound an unborn child hears. When it is finally stilled, it means the end of life.

Rheumatic heart disease may damage its valves. Bacteria can invade its muscle. When the minerals sodium, phosphorus and potassium are out of balance, they can disrupt the heart's electrical activity. The channels of the coronary arteries can become crusted and clogged. But none of this is inevitable. With what we already know, we can take steps to protect ourselves against heart disease. Why not adopt a healthful lifestyle before a heart attack strikes?

No one really argues against the advice to select a well-balanced diet, to cut down on salt and sugar and fat. No one argues against having his blood pressure tested and lowering it if it is too high. No one has found any health benefits from smoking cigarettes. No one claims that exercise is bad for the heart.

Heart disease won't disappear without our help.

• Have your cholesterol measured if you are worried about heart disease or if you have a family history of heart disease.

• Have your blood pressure checked, and take your pills if your doctor prescribes them.

• Find enough time to exercise.

• Find time to relax.

• Eat moderately from a variety of the four food groups: dairy products; grains and cereals; fruits and vegetables; fish, meat and poultry.

• Go to your physician if you have chest pain or find you are easily or suddenly fatigued.

• Watch your weight.

• Seek medical attention if you sense any disturbance in your heart's rhythm.

• Don't smoke; it robs your heart of oxygen.

• Don't count on magic cures; medical miracles are few and far apart.

• Don't believe that it can't happen to you; statistics don't play favorites.

• Don't ignore your body when there is a change in it; it's trying to tell you something.

GLOSSARY

A

angina pectoris
Chest pain due to inadequate oxygenation of heart muscle.

aorta
The main artery arising from the heart.

arrhythmia
A general term for an irregularity in the heartbeat.

arteriosclerosis
A disease of arteries in which deposits of cholesterol and other substances in the artery wall may impede the flow of blood.

artery
Any of a number of blood vessels that carry blood away from the heart to tissues throughout the body.

artificial pacemaker
An electrical device that initiates the heartbeat.

atherosclerosis
A type of arteriosclerosis that first develops beneath the inner wall of an artery.

atrioventricular node   Specialized muscle fibers at the base of the wall between the heart's two upper chambers. These act as a relay in conducting the impulse that generates the heart's beat from the atria to the ventricles.

atrium   One of two upper chambers of the heart.

autonomic nervous system   Nerves that control such functions as the regulation of the heartbeat and the pressure at which the blood flows, as well as myriad other activities in the body that are not under conscious control.

B

blood pressure   The force of the blood against the arteries. See *hypertension*.

C

capillary   The smallest type of blood vessels, in which the transfer of oxygen and nutrients to cells takes place.

cardiac arrest   The cessation of the heartbeat.

cardiopulmonary resuscitation (CPR)   A combination of mouth-to-mouth breathing and heart massage that is performed to sustain the circulation of the blood in a person whose heart is beating ineffectively or in cardiac arrest.

carotid sinus   A small cluster of cells in the carotid arteries that monitors the oxygen and carbon-dioxide content of the blood.

cholesterol   A fatlike substance manufactured by animal cells.

coronary arteries The blood vessels that supply the heart muscle with oxygen and nutrients.

coronary bypass A surgical procedure in which one or more diseased portions of the coronary arteries are tied off and nondiseased vessels, taken from elsewhere in the body, are grafted above and below the blockage to keep the heart muscle supplied with blood and nutrients.

coronary occlusion An obstruction in a coronary artery, shutting off the flow of blood to a portion of the heart muscle. Also called *heart attack* or *myocardial infarction*.

D

defibrillator An electrical device that delivers a shock to the heart.

diastole The phase of the heart's cycle in which the ventricles fill and during which the heart rests for a split second. (This is the "below" number in a blood-pressure reading.)

digitalis A drug, derived from the foxglove plant, used to stimulate the heart.

diuretic A type of medication used to promote the excretion of urine; often given to treat heart failure.

E

electrocardiogram (EKG or ECG)
The graph of sharp peaks and valleys, usually recorded on a strip of paper, of the heart's electrical impulses, and used to help diagnose heart disease.

endocardium
The thin tissue layer of the inner lining of the heart, in contact with the blood.

epicardium
The layer of muscle tissue on the outside of the heart, but just inside the pericardium.

H

heart attack
The death of a portion of the heart muscle. See *myocardial infarction*.

heart block
A condition in which the electrical impulse that coordinates the heartbeat is slowed or blocked along its pathway.

heart failure
A condition in which the heart is unable to pump its required amount of blood; also known as *congestive heart failure*.

heart-lung machine
A device into which the bloodstream is diverted during surgery on or inside the heart. The device adds oxygen to the blood, extracts waste gases, and pumps the blood back into the body to support basic life functions while the heart is stilled.

heart murmur
An abnormal sound emanating from the heart.

hemoglobin
An iron-and-protein complex within red blood cells that carries oxygen.

high-density lipoprotein (HDL)
A normal component of the blood that transports cholesterol.

hormone
Any of a number of normally produced substances secreted into the bloodstream by glands.

hypercholesteremia
An excess of cholesterol in the blood.

hypertension
High blood pressure.

I

insufficiency
Used in conjunction with a specific valve; the incomplete closing of a valve, permitting backflow of blood—as in "mitral insufficiency."

L

low-density lipoprotein (LDL)
A normal component of the blood which transports cholesterol.

lymphocytes
White blood cells; these are involved in manufacturing antibodies and producing immunity.

M

mitral valve
Two specialized leaves of tissue between the left atrium and left ventricle, permitting a one-way flow of blood between those chambers.

myocardial infarction (MI)
The death by interruption of the blood supply of a portion of the heart muscle; the term is sometimes used as a synonym for "heart attack."

myocardium
The muscle of the heart comprising the bulk of the organ, as opposed to the thin tissue that lines the heart's inner and outer surfaces.

N

nitroglycerin
A type of drug used to relieve angina pectoris, or chest pain.

P

pericardium
For *peri* = around, *cardium* = heart; the tough, fibrous sac that surrounds the heart.

plasma
The pale, amber-colored fluid portion of the blood.

R

red blood cells
Doughnut-shaped cells that circulate in the bloodstream carrying oxygen to the cells and the lungs. Also called erythrocytes, or red corpuscles.

rheumatic heart disease
A condition that may result from an untreated streptococcal infection in which the valves of the heart become scarred and progressively less functional.

S

sinoatrial node

A specialized section of modified heart muscle which generates the impulse that causes the heart to beat or contract. Also known as the *pacemaker.*

stenosis

The narrowing of a valve opening in the heart. The term is usually used to describe the condition of the affected valve, as in "mitral stenosis" or "aortic stenosis."

stroke

A blockage in the blood supply to a part of the brain. Also called *cerebrovascular accident.* (Note: A stroke is *not* a type of heart attack.)

systole

The phase of the heart's cycle in which contraction occurs. (This is the "above" number in a blood-pressure reading.)

T

tachycardia

An abnormally fast heartbeat rate at rest.

thrombosis

The formation of a blood clot within a blood vessel. When this happens within a coronary artery it is called *coronary thrombosis* and is synonymous with a heart attack.

tricuspid valve

Three specialized triangular leaves of tissue between the right atrium and right ventricle which open to permit the blood to flow in one direction, from atrium to ventricle, and close to prevent backflow.

V

valve
Two or more flaps of tissue which prevent the backflow of blood; usually used in conjunction with a specific valve, as in "mitral valve" or "tricuspid valve."

vein
Any of a number of blood vessels that carry blood back to the heart.

ventricular fibrillation
A rapid, uncoordinated beat, or arrhythmia, which can be fatal if not corrected within minutes after it begins.

ventricle
One of the two lower chambers of the heart, which are the main pumping chambers.

INDEX

About the Authors

DOUGLAS GASNER, a free-lance writer who is based in New York City, is the former editor of *Psychology Today*. He has been science news editor for the American Medical Association and a medical correspondent for *Time* magazine. Mr. Gasner has written a number of books on medical and scientific topics. He is married and has two children.

ELLIOTT H. MCCLEARY is a professional writer and editor with a special interest in medicine and health. He has served as the editor of *Today's Health* magazine, as senior editor of adult nonfiction for Rand McNally publishers, has written for leading national magazines, and is the author of the book *New Miracles of Childbirth*. He is a member and former Midwest chairman of the American Society of Journalists and Authors.